Laboratory Activities for Therapeutic Modalities

Laboratory Activities for Therapeutic Modalities

Chad Starkey, PhD, ATC
Northeastern University
Boston, MA

Sara D. Brown, MS, ATC
Boston University
Boston, MA

F. A. DAVIS COMPANY · Philadelphia

F. A. Davis Company
1915 Arch Street
Philadelphia, PA 19103

Printed in the United States of America

Last digit indicates print number: 10 9 8 7 6 5 4 3 2 1

Publisher, Allied Health: Jean-François Vilain
Editorial Manager: Rose Gabbay
Cover Designer: Steve Morrone

As new scientific information becomes available through basic and clinical research, recommended treatments and drug therapies undergo changes. The authors and publisher have done everything possible to make this book accurate, up to date, and in accord with accepted standards at the time of publication. The authors, editors, and publisher are not responsible for errors or omissions or for consequences from application of the book, and make no warranty, expressed or implied, in regard to the contents of the book. Any practice described in this book should be applied by the reader in accordance with professional standards of care used in regard to the unique circumstances that may apply in each situation. The reader is advised always to check product information (package inserts) for changes and new information regarding dose and contraindications before administering any drug. Caution is especially urged when using new or infrequently ordered drugs.

Dedication

To my Science Fiction Twin
cas

To Maggie, Mia, Natalie, Jake, their parents, grandparents, and Tom
sdb

The modalities included in the exercises in this laboratory manual are intended to be used according to the manufacturers' safety and operating recommendations. Contraindications to the use of these modalities must be ascertained and observed.

Preface

After many combined years between us of teaching therapeutic modalities, we found a need for structured laboratory activities beyond the rote setup and application of the equipment. Too often students were becoming technicians rather than clinicians. We also found a secondary need to expose the student to the physical sensations and the physiological effects of the energy delivered by therapeutic modalities, reinforcing the didactic segment of our courses. This manual represents our combined efforts to improve the students' laboratory experience with therapeutic modalities.

This laboratory manual is designed to be an adjunctive tool for most of the existing textbooks on therapeutic modalities and should not be considered a stand-alone text on this topic. While we have included contraindications for each of the modalities used (Appendix I), the ultimate responsibility for the safe setup and application rests with the students and their instructors.

While structured procedures are described for each of the activities, they may be modified by the instructor to make use of the available equipment and fit the educational level of the students. Depending on the experience of the student, this laboratory manual provides avenues for incorporating therapeutic exercise into many of the activities, exercises, and case studies. The quasi-experimental design of the activities allows the integration of statistical analysis. Before the beginning of the class, the instructor should refer to Appendix A for an explanation of the equipment used in measuring skin temperature.

Each activity is followed by a series of discussion questions. A brief explanation and rationale for the correct response appears in Appendix E. Perforated pages are provided so that the results of the class activities and exercises can be submitted at the instructor's request. Copies of the grids for each activity are provided in Appendix H. The intent of these grids is to allow the student to repeat an exercise. Please avoid the temptation to copy these for mass distribution.

The manual concludes with a series of case studies. After much deliberation we decided to include only a list of the problems that should be surmised from each case (Appendix G). The wide range of methodologies and ideologies surrounding treatment options made even an effort to create a "correct" response dubious at best.

Chad Starkey
Sara D. Brown

Class Activity 1

Skin Temperature Decrease

Objective: The student will evaluate the relative effectiveness of various cold modalities in decreasing the skin surface temperature and the duration of the decrease.

Materials Needed:

- Surface temperature gauge (Appendix A)
- Various methods of delivering cold (crushed ice bag, ice immersion bucket in the range of 45° to 55°F, ice massage cup, reusable cold pack, instant cold pack, vapocoolant spray)
- Timing device

Procedures:

1. Using the surface temperature gauge, record the baseline skin temperature of the surface area to be evaluated. Record this reading on the chart provided and, using a straightedge, mark this line across the grid. This is your baseline.
2. Apply the cold modality to the body part in the prescribed manner for a total of 10 minutes, with the exception of the vapocoolant spray, which should be applied as recommended by the manufacturer.
3. On removing the modality, measure the skin temperature and record this at the "10-minute" mark on the chart.
4. Every 2 minutes, re-measure the skin temperature and make the proper notation on the chart.
5. Repeat step 4 until the skin temperature returns to the baseline value.
6. Using a different body area on a different extremity, repeat steps 1 through 5 with another cold modality.
7. On completion of the activity, plot the changes in skin temperature resulting from each modality.

Notes:

- This activity may be performed using more than one modality at once provided each is applied to a separate body area.
- If an electronic skin temperature probe is available the changes in skin temperature during the cold application may be measured and recorded in 2-minute intervals.
- A layer of wet insulation must be used when applying reusable cold packs to the body.

Discussion:

The magnitude of skin temperature decrease is directly related to the temperature of the applied modality, the duration of application, and the conductivity of the tissue being cooled. Because the heat transfer is occurring via conduction (or evaporation in the case of the vapocoolant spray), the greater the temperature decrease, the greater the transfer of thermal energy and subsequent cooling of the skin.

Skin Temperature Decrease (Cont.)

Generally, however, cold modalities are used to effect changes deep within the tissues. How does a drop in surface temperature correspond with deep tissue changes? The correlation between the decrease in skin temperature and the decrease in intra-articular temperature has been calculated to be .65.[1] However, the conductivity of the tissues being treated and the duration of the cold application must be considered. Tissues with a low water content, such as fat, are good insulators and do not allow the transfer of thermal energy. (Witness the blubber-protected whale swimming comfortably in the cold ocean.) By comparison, muscle tissue with its relatively high water content is a good conductor and allows the energy to be absorbed and transmitted to deeper tissues. The application duration also influences the depth of penetration. While it does not take long to evoke superficial changes in temperature (as you have just experienced), targeting deep tissues requires a longer application time.

Activity Questions:

1. Of the different types of cold application used, which had the greatest change in surface temperature? Why?

2. If cold acts as a vasoconstrictor, why does the skin turn red during cold application?

3. Based on the skin temperature changes, which method would you assume had the least depth of penetration? How would this influence your selection of a cold modality?

Skin Temperature Decrease Worksheet

Name: ______________________ Date: ____________

Partner(s): ____

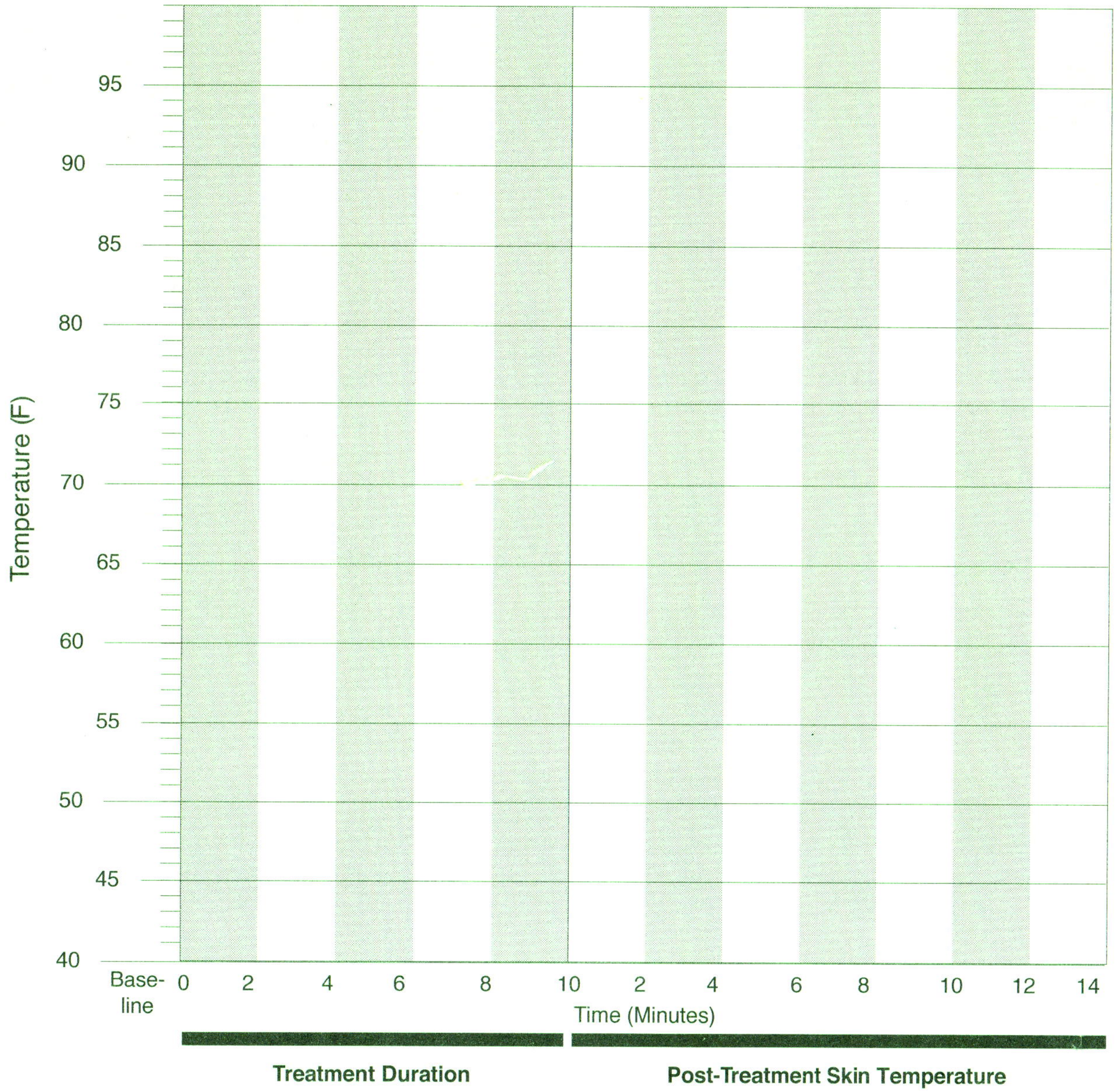

Labeling Key			
○	Crushed Ice Bag	△	Instant Cold Pack
●	Ice Immersion	▲	Vapocoolant Spray
□	Ice Massage	X	Other:
■	Reusable Cold Pack		Other:

Class Activity 2

Pain Perception During Ice Immersion

Objective: The student will gain an understanding of the four sensations commonly related to cold application, aquire knowledge in the use of pain scales, and ascertain the effect of Neoprene™ toe caps in increasing the comfort level of ice immersion.

Materials Needed:
- Ice immersion bucket
- Numerical rating scale
- Neoprene™ toe cap
- Timing device
- Thermometer for measuring the temperature of the immersion

Description of the Numerical Rating Scale:

Several simple pain rating scales may be used to measure an individual's pain objectively. The Visual Analog Scale (VAS) employs a 10-cm line describing a continuum between "no pain," at the low end and the "worst pain imaginable" at the high end (Fig. 1). Subjects mark a point on the line that best represents the current level of pain they are experiencing. The disadvantage of this system is that the lack of coordinates decreases the specificity of rating.[2] The advantage of this system is found in the use of words to describe the extremes of pain.

Figure 1. The Visual Analog Scale (VAS) for rating pain.

The Numerical Rating Scale (NRS) uses a numerical scale ranging from "0," representing "no pain" to "10," representing the "worst pain imaginable." Subjects are then asked to circle the whole number between 0 and 10 that best represents their current pain level. The advantage of this system lies in the use of graded intervals to measure pain intensity. The disadvantage is in the lack of descriptors at the extremes. For use in this workbook we have merged the two scales, combining the intervals of the NRS with the descriptors found in the VAS (Fig. 2).

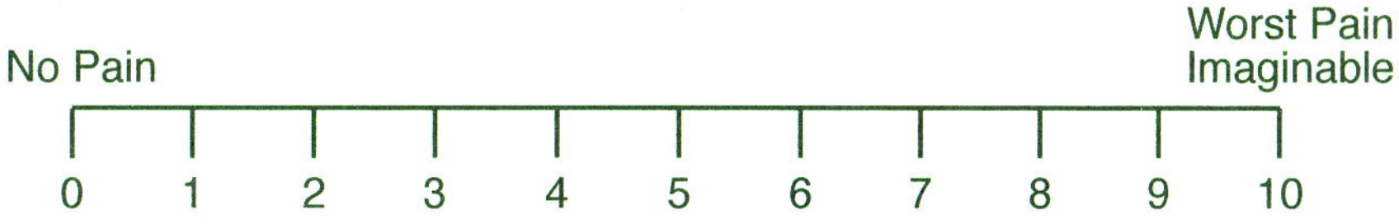

Figure 2. The Numerical Rating Scale (NRS) for measuring pain. This scale has been modified by the authors for use in this workbook by adding the labels "No Pain" and "Worst Pain Imaginable."

Procedures for Using the Numerical Rating Scale

Subjects view the modified NRS and circle the number best describing their current level of pain. It is customary to circle only a whole number. Therefore circling "7" is an appropriate response whereas marking the position on the grid representing "7.5" is not appropriate. When multiple measures are being made, the subject is not permitted to view the previous response. We recommend that once a scale is marked, it be covered with a piece of paper until the exercise is completed.

Procedures:

1. Fill an immersion bucket with water and add enough ice to decrease the temperature between 50° and 55°F.
2. Inform the subject that this activity will cause a moderate amount of pain. If the pain becomes too great or if the subject experiences lightheadedness, discontinue the activity.
3. Instruct the subject to immerse a leg in the bucket.
4. After 1 minute have the subject circle the number on the modified NRS that best describes the level of pain experienced.
5. Cover this and future responses so that the subject cannot see the previous responses.
6. Repeat the pain scale every 2 minutes for the duration of the treatment.
7. Plot the changes in perception of cold sensation over time on the accompanying worksheet.
8. Repeat this activity with the same subject using the opposite leg. However, this time have the subject cover the toes with a Neoprene™ toe cap.

Discussion:

The degree of vulnerability of different nerves to cold application accounts for the changes in sensation experienced as the cold treatment progresses. Unmyelinated, small-diameter, superficial pain nerves are stimulated before the larger, myelinated, and deeper lying nerves. The initial pain experienced during ice immersion results from stimulation of pain-carrying nerves. As the exposure to the cold continues, the perception of pain decreases because of the decrease in nerve conduction velocity of these nerves and the subsequent stimulation of sensory nerves.

It is commonly reported that four distinct sensory phases will be experienced during cold application: cold, burning, aching, and analgesia.[3] However, true anesthesia (the inability to transmit nerve impulses) has not been proven to occur during ice immersion.[4]

Activity Questions:

1. Did your foot and ankle become numb during the immersion?

2. Most people, especially first-time cold users, find this exercise painful. Where was your pain primarily located? Did the use of the toe cap change your perception of pain? Repeat this activity a week later. How do your responses vary?

Pain Perception During Ice Immersion Worksheet

Name: ______________________ Date: ____________

Partner(s): ______________________________________

1 Minute Post-Immersion

No Pain — Worst Pain Imaginable

0 1 2 3 4 5 6 7 8 9 10

3 Minutes Post-Immersion

No Pain — Worst Pain Imaginable

0 1 2 3 4 5 6 7 8 9 10

5 Minutes Post-Immersion

No Pain — Worst Pain Imaginable

0 1 2 3 4 5 6 7 8 9 10

7 Minutes Post-Immersion

No Pain — Worst Pain Imaginable

0 1 2 3 4 5 6 7 8 9 10

9 Minutes Post-Immersion

No Pain — Worst Pain Imaginable

0 1 2 3 4 5 6 7 8 9 10

11 Minutes Post-Immersion

No Pain — Worst Pain Imaginable

0 1 2 3 4 5 6 7 8 9 10

Plot of Pain Perception Over Time

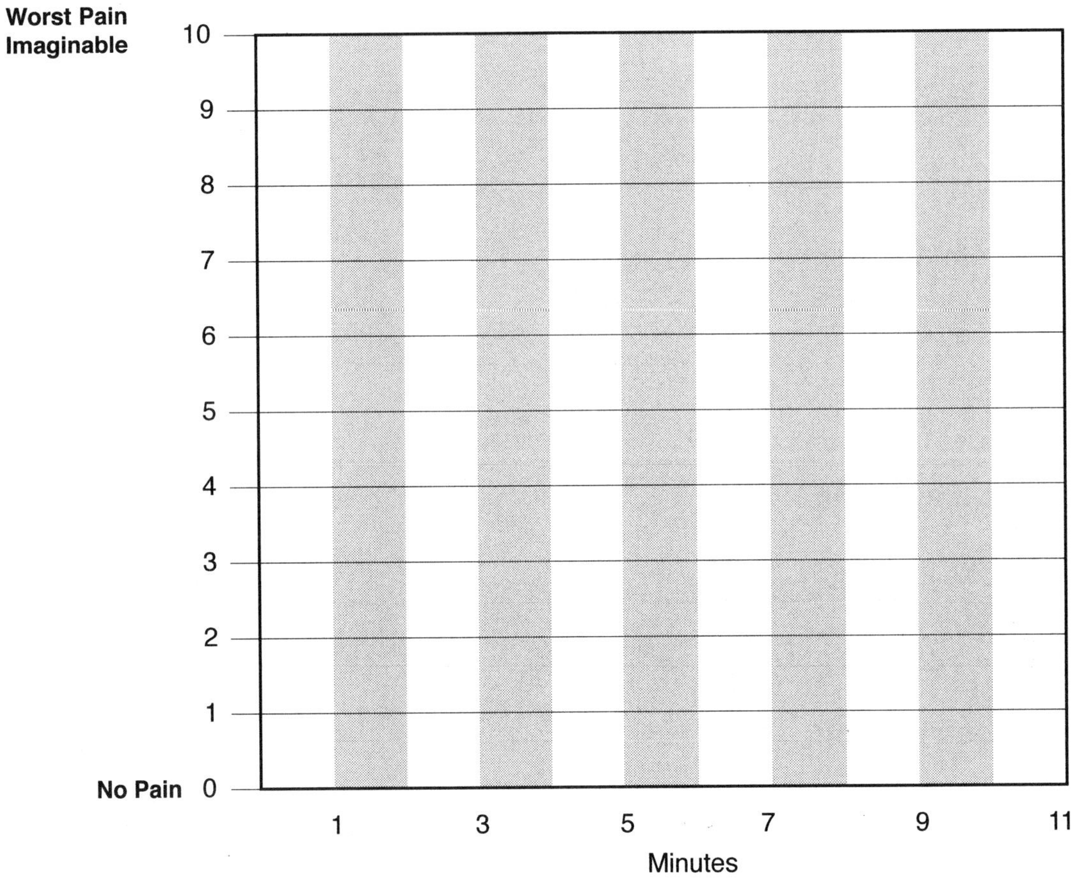

Labeling Key	
■	No Toe Cap
●	With Toe Cap

Class Activity 3

Effects of Insulating Media on Skin Temperature Decrease

Objective: The student will determine the effect that various insulating media have on the rate and magnitude of skin temperature decrease.

Materials Needed:

- Crushed ice pack
- Wet elastic wrap
- Thermometer
- Damp terry cloth towel
- Dry terry cloth towel
- Timing device

Procedures:

1. Using the surface temperature gauge, record the baseline skin temperature of the area to be treated. Record this reading on the chart provided and, using a straight-edge, mark this line across the grid.
2. Cover the area to be treated with an insulating medium and apply the crushed ice pack for a total of 10 minutes.
3. On removing the modality, measure the skin temperature and record this at the "10-minute" mark on the chart.
4. Every 2 minutes, remeasure the skin temperature and make the proper notation on the chart.
5. Repeat step 4 until the skin temperature returns to the baseline value.
6. Using a different body area on a different extremity, repeat steps 1 through 5 with a different form of insulation.
7. On completion of the activity, plot the changes in skin temperature resulting from each modality. To obtain an estimate of the decrease in temperature drop, transpose the skin temperature decrease for a crushed ice pack, obtained during Class Activity 1, if completed, onto this grid.

Notes:

- This activity may be performed using more than one cold treatment at once provided each is applied to a separate body area.
- If an electronic skin temperature probe is available, the changes in skin temperature during the cold application may be measured and recorded in 2-minute intervals.

Discussion:

The fear of frostbite causes many clinicians to apply an insulator such as an ace wrap or towel between the cold modality and the skin. Does this practice reduce the effectiveness of the treatment? Because a relationship exists between reduction in skin temperature and the temperature reduction in tissues underlying the treatment area, by measuring the reduction in surface temperature under different treatment conditions, we can ascertain the relative effectiveness of different treatment techniques.

Effects of Insulating Media on Skin Temperature Decrease (Cont.)

The risk of frostbite depends on the temperature of the applied modality, the duration of the treatment, and the neurovascular properties of the area being treated. Cold modalities that use frozen water, crushed ice packs, ice massage, or ice immersion have a decreased risk of tissue damage because of the melting of the ice. When these cold modalities are applied to a body part that has intact nervous and vascular function for the recommended treatment duration (10 to 30 minutes), the chance of frostbite is virtually nonexistent, even when the modality is applied directly to the skin. However, when a modality such as a reusable cold pack (which is water mixed with antifreeze and stored at temperatures well below the freezing point) is used or when cold modalities are applied for an extended duration, the chance of frostbite increases. For this reason, reusable cold packs must be applied with a wet insulating medium. The risk of frostbite also increases when cold is applied to areas with poor neurovascular function. When using cold modalities on individuals with conditions such as peripheral vascular disease, the skin must be insulated and the individual closely monitored.

Activity Questions:

1. Considering the relationship between tissue water content and conductivity discussed in Class Activity 1, under which condition would you expect the greatest surface temperature change?

2. What can you conclude about the effectiveness of ice application using different insulating media?

Effects of Insulating Media on Skin Temperature Decrease Worksheet

Name: ____________________ Date: ____________

Partner(s): ________________________________

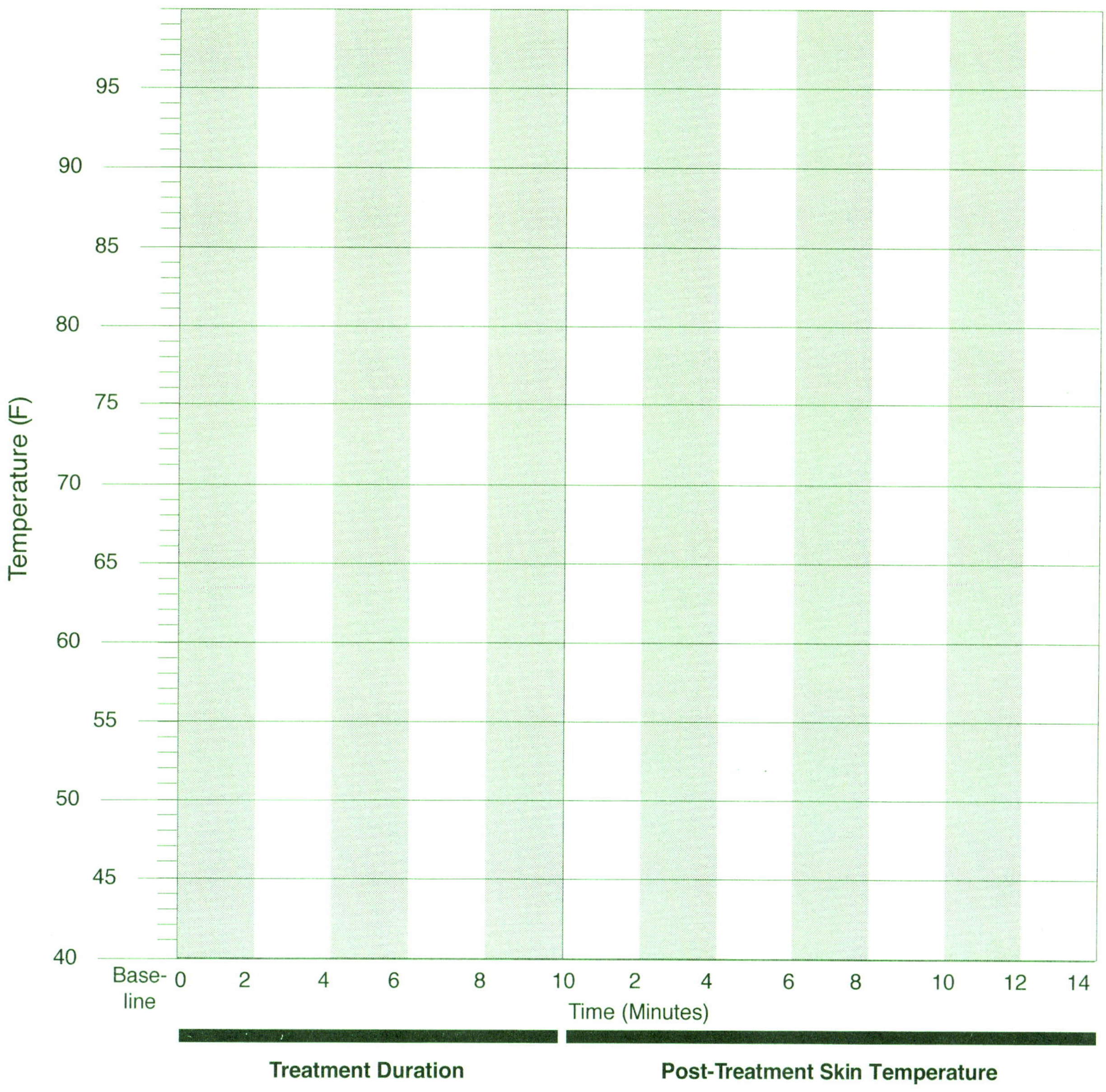

Labeling Key

Symbol	Medium	Symbol	Medium
○	Wet Elastic Wrap	■	No Insulation (From Activity 1)
●	Dry Terry Cloth	△	Other
□	Damp Terry Cloth	▲	Other

Class Activity 4

Skin Temperature Increase

Objective: The student will determine the relative effectiveness of various heat modalities in increasing the skin surface temperature and the duration of the increase.

Materials Needed:
- Surface temperature gauge
- Timing device

Various methods of delivering heat:
- Moist heat pack
- Paraffin
- Warm whirlpool
- Moist heat pack
- Infrared lamp

Procedures:

1. Using the surface temperature gauge, record the baseline skin temperature of the area to be treated. Record this reading on the chart provided and, using a straightedge, mark this line across the grid.
2. Apply the heat modality to the body part in the prescribed manner for a total of 10 minutes.
3. On removing the modality, measure the skin temperature and record this at the "10-minute" mark on the chart.
4. Remeasure the skin temperature at 2 minute intervals and make the proper notation on the chart.
5. Repeat step 4 until the skin temperature returns to the baseline value.
6. Using a different body area on a different extremity, repeat steps 1 through 5 with a different modality.
7. On completion of the activity, plot the changes in skin temperature resulting from each modality.

Notes:

- This activity may be performed using more than one modality at once provided each is applied to a separate body area.
- If an electronic skin temperature probe is available the changes in skin temperature during the heat application may be measured and recorded in 2 minute intervals.
- A counterirritant agent may be used to demonstrate its effect on skin temperature.

Discussion:

As with the application of cold, the surface temperature increase with application of a heat modality correlates to the subcutaneous temperature increase. The extent of the surface temperature increase depends on the treatment duration and the conductive qualities of the heating agent. In general, heat does not penetrate as deeply as cold because the increased blood flow acts to dissipate the heat.

Activity Questions:

1. Which of the modalities used demonstrated the greatest skin temperature increase?

2. Compare the findings of the skin temperature increase and the skin temperature decrease exercises. Which condition demonstrated the longer time for return to normal skin temperature? Why does this occur?

Skin Temperature Increase Worksheet

Name: ______________________ Date: ______________

Partner(s): ______________________________________

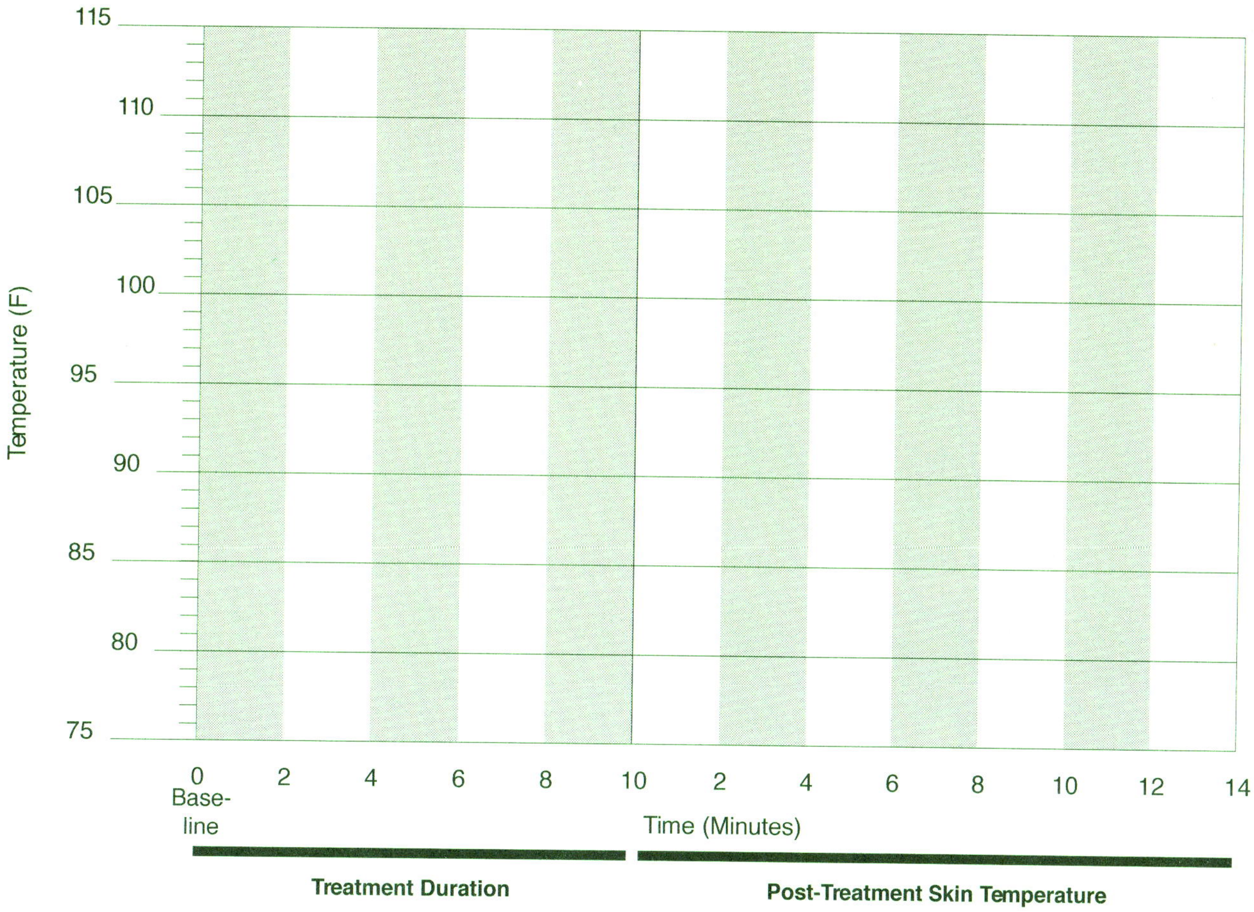

Labeling Key

○	Moist Heat Pack	■	Warm Water Immersion
●	Dry Heat	△	Other
□	Paraffin	▲	Other

Class Activity 5

Effect of Heat and Cold on Tissue Elasticity

Objective: The student will determine the effect of heat and cold application has on tissue elasticity and joint range of motion (ROM).

Materials Needed:
- Ice pack
- Moist heat pack
- Method of determining hamstring flexibility (see discussion below)

Measurement of Hamstring Flexibility

Several methods may be used to determine the flexibility of the hamstring group. For the purposes of this exercise, the method used must be objective so that the pre-test and post-test scores may be accurately measured. We recommend the use of one of three techniques, although any objective method may be used:

Sit-and-Reach: This method incorporates a measuring device (such as two rulers) that is attached to a box. The subject sits with the knees straight and the feet flat against the box; the measurement at this point is labeled "0." The subject then reaches along the measuring device, and the measurement is taken at the point where the stretch is held. If the subject is unable to reach beyond the bottom of the feet, it is recorded as a negative number and if the subject stretches beyond the feet, it is recorded as a positive value (Fig. 3).

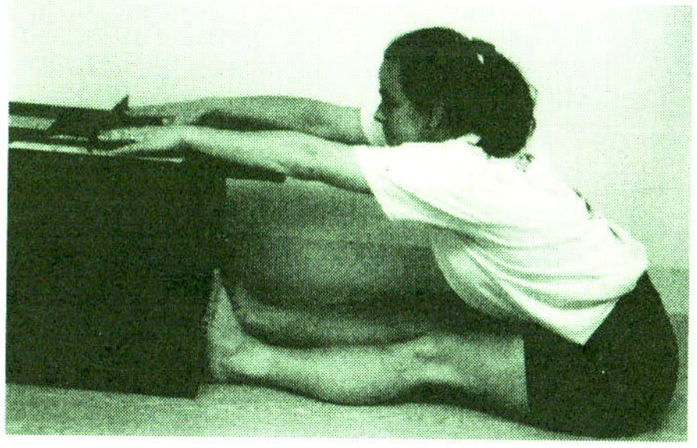

Figure 3. Sit-and-reach technique of measuring hamstring flexibility.

Goniometric Measurement: This method requires the use of a goniometer to assess the amount of hip flexion with the subject's knee kept straight. The measurement is taken with the subject lying supine. Align the stationary arm along the subject's torso so that it is kept parallel with the table top, the axis is aligned with the greater trochanter, and the movement arm aligned with the femoral shaft. The hip is then flexed to its maximal ROM (Fig. 4). Care must be taken to ensure that common reference points are used during all tests and that lumbopelvic motion does not occur.

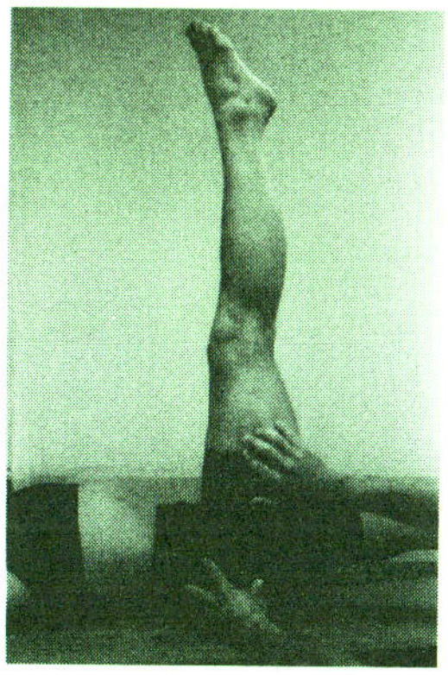

Figure 4. Goniometric evaluation of hip flexion.

Stand-and-Reach: This is the simplest of the three methods. The subject stands with the feet shoulder width apart and the knees straight. The subject then leans over and attempts to touch the palms to the floor (Fig. 5). Using a yardstick or

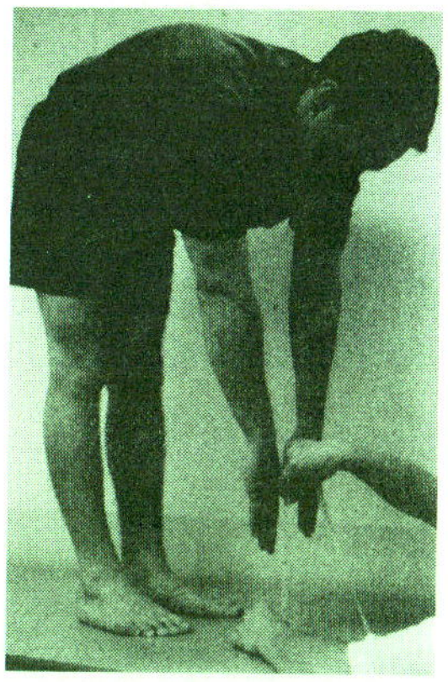

Figure 5. Stand-and-reach method of measuring hamstring flexibility.

Procedures:

1. The instructor may wish to randomly divide the class into two groups, one to receive cold packs and the other to receive heat packs.
2. Determine the baseline amount of hamstring flexibility and record it on the worksheet.
3. Apply the modality (hot or cold) to both hamstring groups using the proper protocol for 10 minutes.
4. Immediately after the termination of the treatment, remeasure the amount of hamstring flexibility and record it on the worksheet.
5. Calculate the net increase or decrease in the range of motion.
6. Using the values obtained by the class, categorize the pre-test/post-test scores using the chart provided.
7. Statistical analysis, such as the t-test , may be used to determine if there is a significant difference between the techniques.

Discussion:

Thermal agents are often used to facilitate soft tissue flexibility and joint ROM. The reasons for choosing cold or heat therapy range from the stage of the injury being treated to the preference of the individual being treated. Cold may be preferred because of its pain-reducing capacity; heat may be selected for its effects on collagen extensibility. Regardless of the choice, the clinician must remember that the modality is only as effective as the therapeutic exercise subsequently used.

Activity Questions:

1. Which treatment condition resulted in the greatest increase in hamstring flexibility?
2. Repeat this activity incorporating a hamstring stretch following the modality application. How does this alter your results?

Effect of Heat and Cold on Tissue Elasticity Worksheet

Name: ______________________ Date: ____________

Partner(s): ____

Hamstring ROM Measurement Used: ☐ Sit-and-Reach ☐ Goniometer ☐ Stand-and-Reach ☐ Other: ____________

Subject	Modality Used	Pre-Test	Post-Test
	☐ Heat ☐ Cold		
	☐ Heat ☐ Cold		
	☐ Heat ☐ Cold		
	☐ Heat ☐ Cold		
	☐ Heat ☐ Cold		

Composite Scores:

Cold Application			
Subject	Pre	Post	Diff
Net Change			

Heat Application			
Subject	Pre	Post	Diff
Net Change			

Class Activity 6

Effect of Heat and Cold on Pulse and Blood Pressure

Objective: The student will determine what, if any, systemic changes occur in pulse and blood pressure resulting from the local application of heat and cold.

Materials Needed:
- Watch with a second hand
- Blood pressure cuff and stethoscope
- Tub of hot or cold water (the range for the hot immersion should range between 98° to 105° F; the cold immersion should range from 45° to 55°F)

Procedures:

1. Using the right arm, determine the subject's pulse rate and blood pressure. To monitor the pulse, palpate the radial artery at the anterior wrist for 15 seconds. and multiply that value by 4 to get the beats per minute. On the first chart, record these baseline values.
2. Immerse the left arm in a tub of hot or cold water.
3. In 2-minute intervals, recheck and record the subject's pulse rate and blood pressure for a total of 10 minutes (Fig. 6).
4. Continue to monitor the pulse and blood pressure until both measures return to their original values or 10 minutes pass.
5. Repeat steps 1 through 4 using the other modality. Record these findings on the second chart.
6. Plot the changes in blood pressure (left vertical axis) and pulse (right vertical axis) using the symbol key provided.

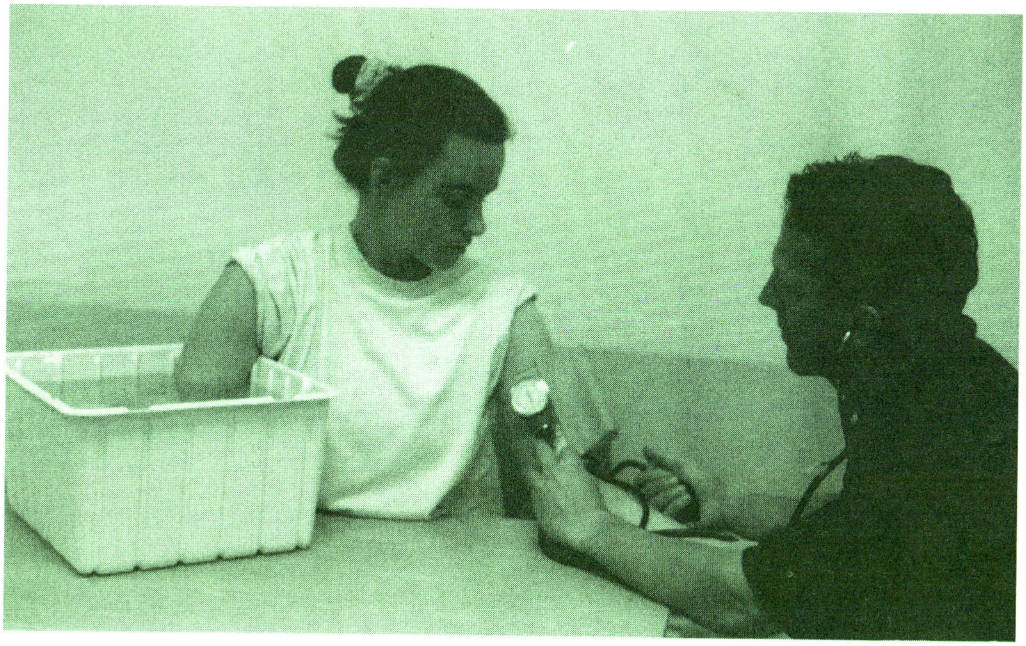

Figure 6. Setup of immersion with blood pressure and pulse assessment.

Discussion:

It is generally accepted that the therapeutic application of cold results in vasoconstriction, whereas the application of heat results in vasodilation. Subsequently, these local vascular events could result in increased systemic blood pressure secondary to vasoconstriction and decreased blood pressure secondary to vasodilation. Additionally, cold exposure cools the hypothalamus, decreasing the pulse rate, whereas heat exposure may result in an increased pulse as the body attempts to cool itself.

The magnitude of these effects largely depends on the temperature gradient and the proportion of the body exposed. As you have just experienced in this activity, the extent of these systemic changes is for all purposes clinically insignificant during localized therapeutic heat or cold treatments.

Activity Questions:

1. What logical contraindications could be derived from this exercise regarding full body immersion in cold or hot water?

2. How would you expect these results to change if a larger proportion of the body were exposed to cold application? To heat application?

Effect of Heat and Cold on Pulse and Blood Pressure Worksheet

Name: ______________________ Date: ______________

Partner(s): ______________________________________

Type of Modality Used: ☐ Heat ☐ Cold

Test Measurements:

	Baseline	During Application					Post-Application				
		2	4	6	8	10	2	4	6	8	10
Pulse											
Blood Pressure	/	/	/	/	/	/	/	/	/	/	/

Plot of Changes in Blood Pressure and Pulse Rate

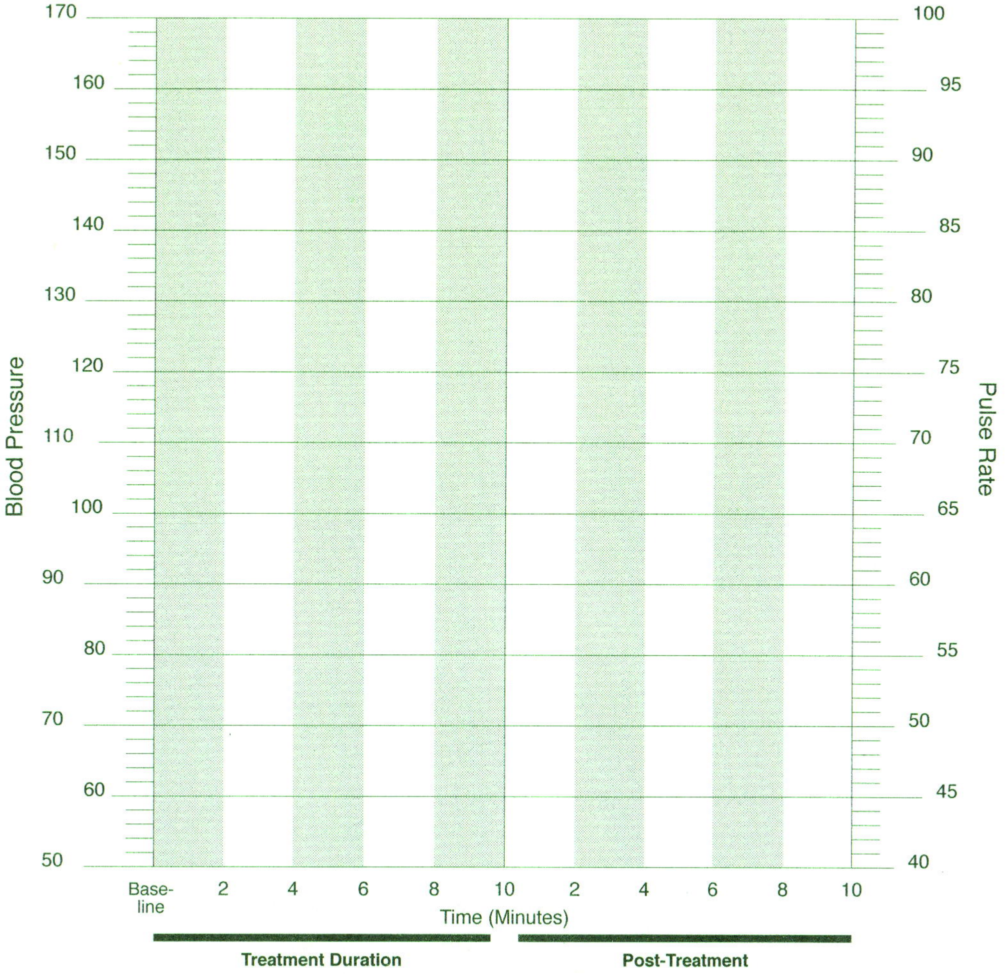

Labeling Key			
Blood Pressure (left axis)			Pulse Rate (right axis)
●	Systolic Pressure	■	Pulse Rate
○	Diastolic Pressure		

Type of Modality Used: ☐ Heat ☐ Cold

Test Measurements:

	Baseline	During Application 2	4	6	8	10	Post-Application 2	4	6	8	10
Pulse											
Blood Pressure											

Plot of Changes in Blood Pressure and Pulse Rate

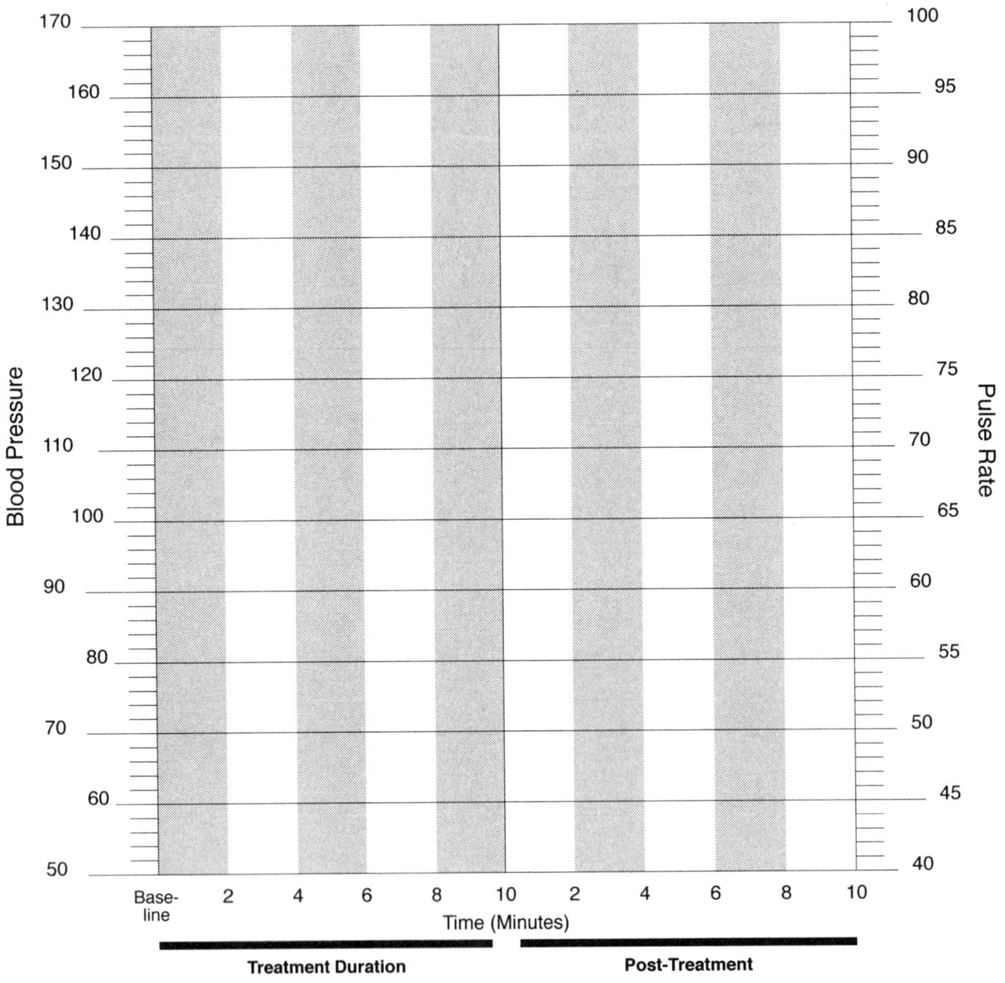

Labeling Key			
Blood Pressure (left axis)			Pulse Rate (right axis)
●	Systolic Pressure	■	Pulse Rate
○	Diastolic Pressure		

Selective Stimulation of Nerves

Objective: Using a strength-duration curve, the student will understand how adjustment of the pulse duration affects the level of intensity required to stimulate sensory, motor, and pain nerve fibers.

Materials Needed: Electrical stimulation unit with an adjustable pulse duration (high-volt pulsed stimulator or neuromuscular electrical stimulation recommended).

Procedures:

1. Depending on the stimulating unit used, select either a monopolar or bipolar electrode configuration. When a monopolar electrode configuration is used, attach the "dispersive" electrode on the subject's lower back or thigh and the "active" electrode to the anterior portion of the subject's forearm (this configuration is recommended for high-volt pulsed units). If other stimulators are used, arrange the electrodes in a bipolar configuration with one electrode being placed on the distal portion of the subject's anterior forearm and the other on the proximal portion of the anterior forearm (Fig. 7).

2. Set the stimulation parameters to the following values:

Pulse Duration:	25 μsec (or lowest possible value)
Pulse Frequency:	30 pps
Pad Alternating Rate:	Continuous
Modulation Parameters:	Off (constant output)
Duty Cycle:	100%
Polarity:	Positive

Note: Not all parameters will apply to each unit.

3. Position the stimulation unit so that the subject cannot see the intensity reading.

4. Slowly increase the intensity to the level where the subject first reports the sensation of electrical current flow. Record the output intensity on the grid provided.

5. Further increase the intensity until a visible muscle contraction can be seen and record the output intensity.

6. Continue to increase the intensity until the subject reports discomfort resulting from the stimulation. Record the output intensity and reduce the intensity to zero.

7. Allow the subject recovery time from the stimulation bout.

8. Repeat steps 3 through 7 using increased pulse durations (e.g., 10 μsec, 20 μsec, 40 μsec, 80 μsec, and 160 μsec).

9. Conclude this activity using the original pulse duration.

10. Plot the changes in the output intensity required to stimulate sensory nerves, motor nerves, and pain nerves between the various pulse durations.

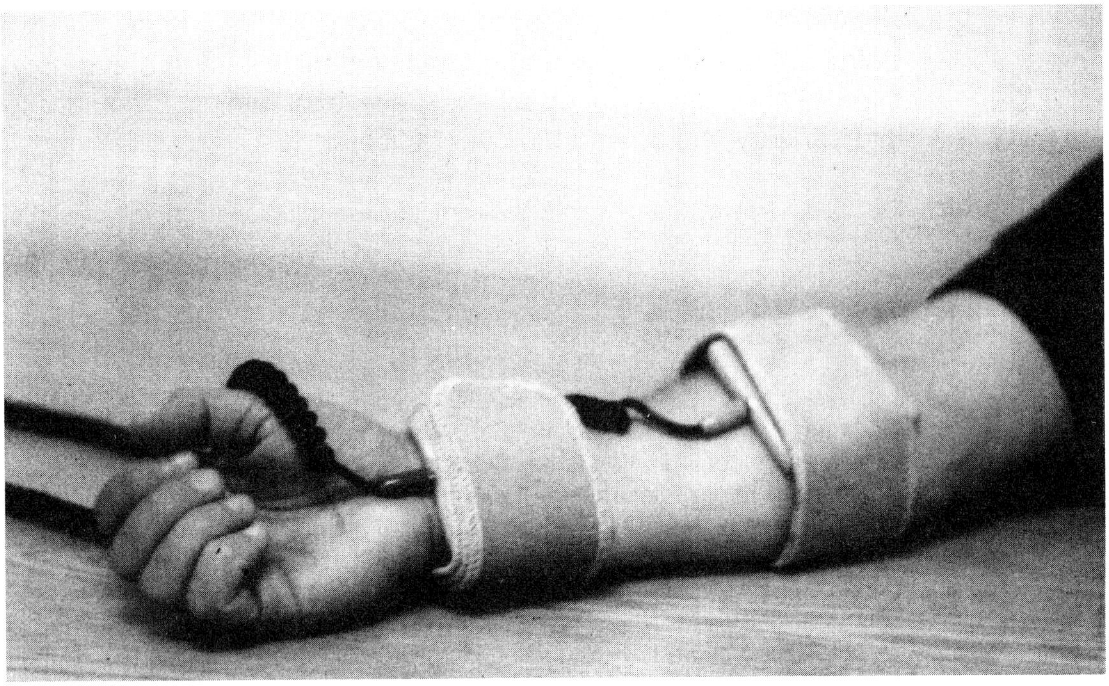

Figure 7. Electrode arrangement for the selective stimulation of nerves.

Discussion:

The use of electrical stimulation incorporates a wide variety of application techniques. Some protocols call for sensory-level stimulation only, whereas others use an electrically induced muscle contraction. Occasionally, even a noxious (painful) stimulus is desired. Each of these sensations results from the response of a particular type of nerve. Whether or not a nerve fires in response to electrical stimulation is determined by the nerve's diameter and depth and by the pulse duration and intensity of the stimulation.

The larger the diameter of the nerve, the lower its resistance and the lower the amplitude necessary for its stimulation. Logically, deeper nerves require a greater amplitude for stimulation than more superficial nerves. In normal, innervated tissue, the order in which nerves are stimulated is constant. As the intensity is increased, sensory fibers are stimulated first, followed by motor nerves, and then pain fibers. If the intensity is allowed to be increased past the point of pain, muscle fibers are then directly stimulated. Short pulse durations allow for the greatest selectivity in the stimulation of these fibers. As the pulse duration is increased, the amount of selectivity between the individual fibers is decreased.

Activity Questions:

1. Was the interval between sensory, motor, and pain stimulation reduced as the pulse duration was increased?

2. Based on your results, what would be the optimal pulse duration if your treatment goal was to achieve maximal sensory stimulation without muscle contraction?

3. Note that the electrode-skin interface will affect resistance. Does the actual amplitude reading have any clinical relevance?

4. Compare the two readings of the shortest pulse duration. Were they the same? To what do you attribute any difference?

Selective Stimulation of Nerves Worksheet

Name: ______________________ Date: ____________

Partner(s): ____

Type of Stimulation Unit Used: ______________________________

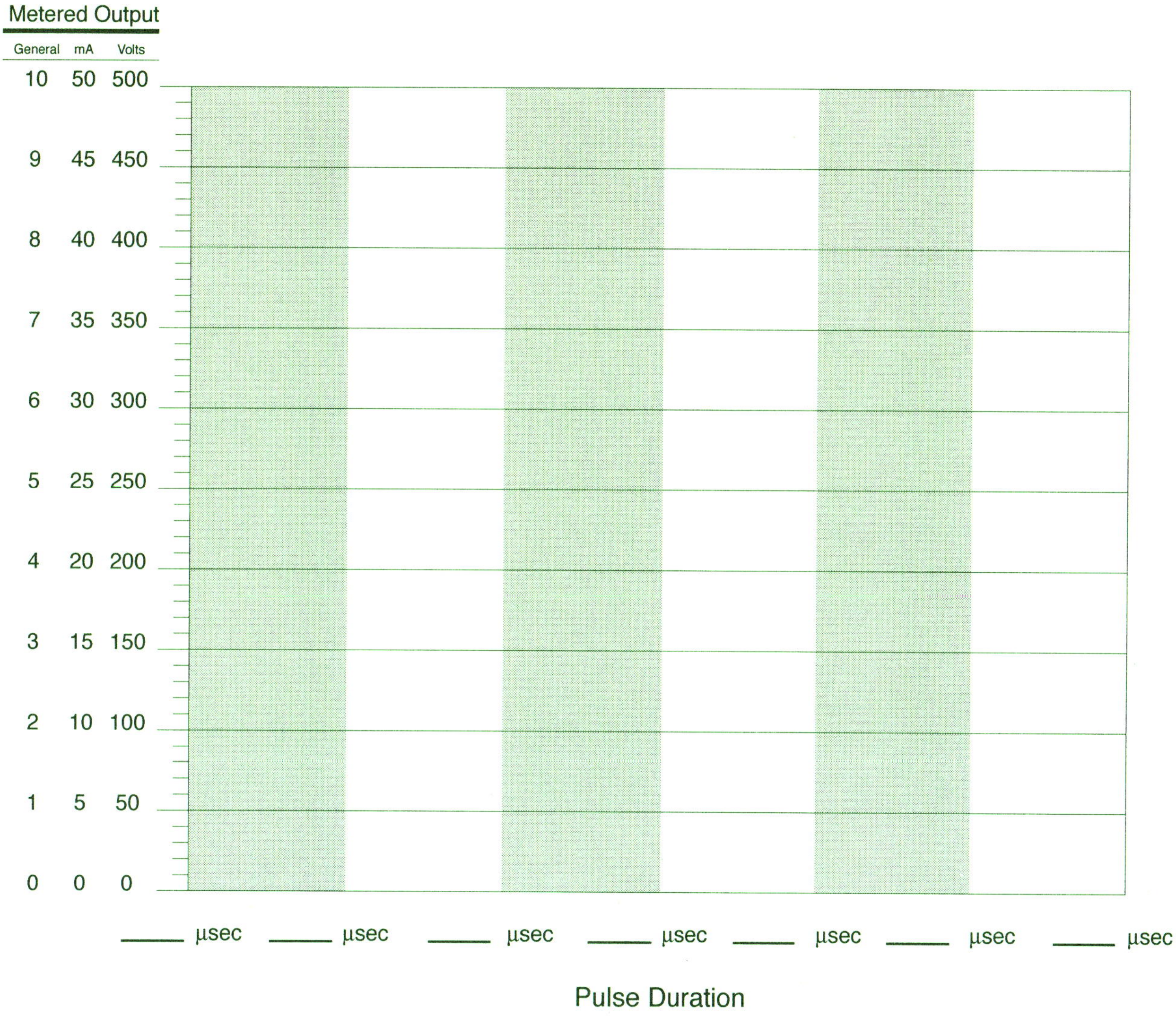

Labeling Key	
●	Sensory Nerves
○	Motor Nerves
□	Pain Nerves

Current Density

Objective: The student will understand the effects of current density on the perception of electrical current flow.

Materials Needed:
- Immersion bucket (filled at least 11 inches deep with warm water)
- Electrical stimulation (ES) unit designed to operate when the electrodes are submerged in water (high-volt pulsed stimulation recommended)

Description of Concurrent Immersion and Electrical Stimulation:

Electrical stimulation may be delivered to a large area by immersing the body part in a tub of water (during therapeutic treatments the temperature of the water is cold for acute injuries and warm/hot for more chronic conditions). One lead, usually a "dispersive" electrode, is attached to the athlete while the active electrode is immersed in the water (Fig. 8). In this configuration, the water touching the immersed extremity (through its length, around its circumference, and around the length and circumference of the phalanges) serves as an interface for conducting the current.

The patient's perception of an electrical current is based on two factors: (1) the intensity of the output and (2) the density of the current under the electrode. Consider a current of 300 volts flowing through an electrode of 10 square inches, the resultant current density would be 30 volts per square inch. If the size of the electrode were reduced to 5 square inches, the current density would be 60 volts per square inch. Assuming that the intensity of the output remains the same, the perception of the stimulus would be greater with the smaller electrodes than with the larger electrodes.

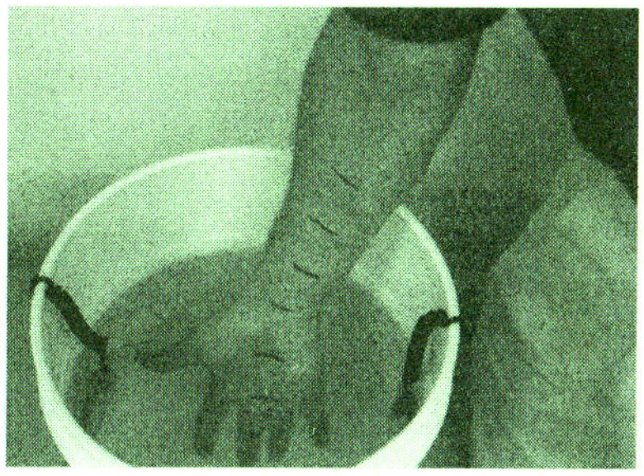

Figure 8. Electrical stimulation during water immersion.

Procedure:

- IT IS IMPORTANT THAT THE SUBJECT DOES NOT COMPLETELY REMOVE THE HAND FROM THE WATER WHILE THE CURRENT IS FLOWING! Please advise your subject of this caveat before proceeding and provide regular reminders throughout this exercise.
- **If the stimulator is operated by standard current, ensure that it is plugged into a ground fault interrupter.**

1. On the subject's nondominant anterior hand and forearm, measure 2 inches proximally from the tip of the middle finger and make a transverse mark. Label this mark "1." Moving proximally in 2-inch increments, mark and label lines "2" through "5" (Fig. 9).
2. Place one or two electrodes in the tub of water and position them so that the rubber insulating material is facing inwards toward the center of the bucket (see Fig. 8).

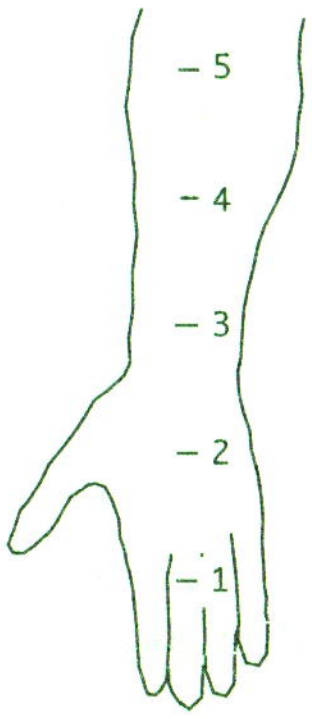

Figure 9. Increments marked on the anterior arm and hand.

3. Instruct the subject not to touch the electrodes or the stimulation unit at any time during this exercise.
4. With the subject seated, fasten a large dispersive electrode to the subject's thigh on the same side as the active electrode. The subject's arm will be immersed in the water in a later step.
5. Set the stimulation parameters to the following values:

Pulse Duration:	25 to 50 μsec
Pulse Frequency:	100 pps
Pad Alternating Rate:	Continuous
Modulation Parameters:	Off (constant output)
Duty Cycle:	100%

Note: Not all parameters will apply to each unit.

6. Make sure that the output intensity is reduced to zero.
7. Instruct the subject to immerse the arm in the water to the "5" mark. For safety, remind the subject again not to completely remove the arm from the water while the current is flowing. When an intensity is too great, instruct the subject to reimmerse the arm, not withdraw it.
8. Slowly increase the intensity to the level where the subject first experiences the sensation of an electrical current. Using the Numerical Rating Scale, have the subject record the perceived intensity of the stimulus. Cover this and future responses to prevent them from influencing the subject's subsequent ratings.
9. Instruct the subject to gradually withdraw the arm to the "4" mark and record the perceived intensity of the stimulus.
10. Repeat the same sequence so that the subject moves to the "3," "2," and "1" mark and record the perceived stimulus for each. Note that some subjects will not be able to tolerate the stimulus at the "2" or "1" levels. If this is case, have the subject record the perception of the tolerable stimulus, reduce the intensity to zero and conclude the activity.

Discussion:

This activity illustrates electricity's tendency to take the path of least resistance and the need to have an adequate conducting medium when using electrical stimulation. As described above, the surface of the submerged hand is analogous to the body surface under an electrode. The submerged hand, however, will always be wet and thus provided an unchanging surface area for conducting the electricity. When using electrodes applied directly to the skin with a coupling medium, this is not always the case.

Little or no stimulation is detected under the dispersive pad when using a monopolar pad configuration because the surface area of the dispersive pad is greater than the surface area of the treatment pads. The current density is greater at the pads with the smaller surface area. When the subject shifts off of the dispersive pad during treatment or the conducting medium dries out, a greater current density occurs along this diminished pathway. The perceived sensation increases, sometimes painfully so.

For this reason, gel is often used as a coupling agent instead of water when electrical stimulation is applied over a long period of time. The gels are less apt to dry out and therefore deliver current at a constant density.

Activity Questions:

1. It was emphasized that the subject should not completely remove his or her arm from the immersion bucket while the current was flowing. Why should this be avoided?

2. As you are increasing the current intensity during an ES treatment with a monopolar electrode arrangement, the person describes feeling the current primarily at the dispersive electrode. What steps would you take to have sensory stimulation under the active electrode(s) only?

Current Density Worksheet

Name: ______________________ Date: ____________

Partner(s): ______________________________________

Type of Stimulation Unit Used: ______________________________

Stimulus Perception at the Level "5" Mark

No Sensation — Intolerable Sensation

0 1 2 3 4 5 6 7 8 9 10

Stimulus Perception at the Level "4" Mark

No Sensation — Intolerable Sensation

0 1 2 3 4 5 6 7 8 9 10

Stimulus Perception at the Level "3" Mark

No Sensation — Intolerable Sensation

0 1 2 3 4 5 6 7 8 9 10

Stimulus Perception at the Level "2" Mark

No Sensation — Intolerable Sensation

0 1 2 3 4 5 6 7 8 9 10

Stimulus Perception at the Level "1" Mark

No Sensation — Intolerable Sensation

0 1 2 3 4 5 6 7 8 9 10

Class Activity 9

Identification of Motor Points

Objective: The student will be able to locate and identify motor points for specific muscles.

Materials Needed: Electrical stimulation unit with a hand-held applicator (high-volt pulsed stimulator recommended)

Description of Motor Points:

Motor points are superficial areas on the skin that have decreased resistance to electrical current flow. Stimulation of these sites causes large motor nerves to depolarize and therefore isolates the contraction to a single muscle or portion of a muscle. The exact locations of motor points tend to vary from individual to individual, but their approximate locations have been identified in many motor point charts. Motor points are not to be confused with trigger points, which are hypersensitive areas that develop secondary to trauma (although they do frequently tend to be found in close proximity to each other).

Procedures:

1. Attach the dispersive electrode to the subject's thigh or lower back and configure the stimulation unit to the hand-held applicator mode. On units not having a provision for a hand-held probe, a small (e.g., 2- by 2-inch) electrode may be used. In this case, attach the dispersive electrode to the subject's thigh and manually move the electrode with one hand while controlling the output intensity with the other.

2. Set the stimulation parameters to the following values:

Pulse Duration:	25 to 50 μsec
Pulse Frequency:	50 pps
Pad Alternating Rate:	Continuous
Modulation Parameters:	Off (constant output)
Polarity of the Active Electrode:	Negative
Duty Cycle:	100%

Note: Not all parameters will apply to each unit.

3. The subject should be lying prone on the table for this exercise.

4. Reset the generator's output intensity to zero and wet the applicator's tip with water or gel.

5. Place the applicator tip on the subject's forearm and slowly increase the intensity to where a slight muscle contraction is visible (Fig. 10).

6. Use the applicator tip to identify the point(s) on the skin which result in strong, isolated contractions of the following muscles:

Upper Extremity	Lower Extremity
Abductor pollicis	Abductor digiti minimi
Extensor digiti minimi	Extensor hallucis longus
Extensor indicis	Extensor digitorum brevis
Flexor carpi radialis	Plantaris
Flexor carpi ulnaris	Tibialis anterior

7. The intensity of the stimulation may need to be adjusted as the applicator is moved over the skin. Most applicators have an intensity adjustment knob located on them. Note: When the applicator tip is removed from the skin, reduce the intensity to "zero" before reapplying it to the subject.

8. Using the labeling key, mark the location of each motor point identified on the accompanying charts.

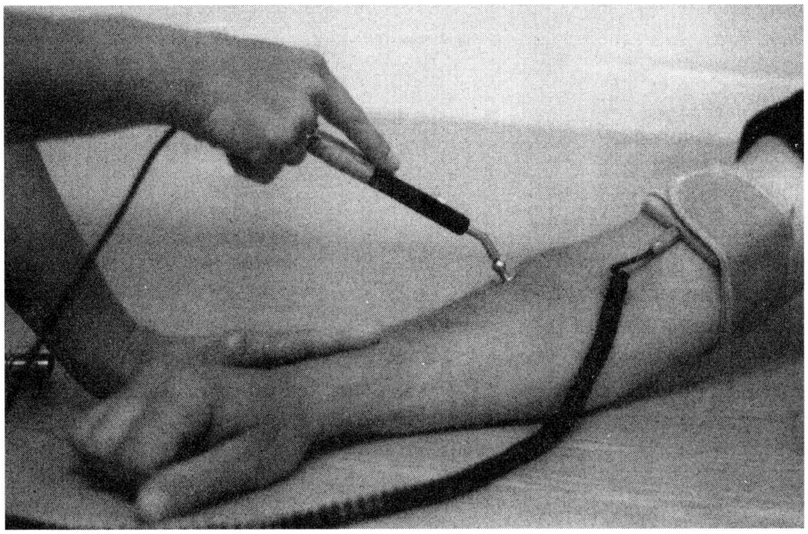

Figure 10. Setup for the identification of motor points using a hand-held applicator.

Discussion:

When using electrical stimulation to elicit a muscular contraction, the placement of the electrodes greatly influences the amount of current necessary to elicit a contraction. Placing the electrodes directly over motor points enables the clinician to produce a maximum motor response using a minimum of current.

In theory, the polarity used (when a choice is possible) can also affect the motor response. According to Pfleuger's law, less current is required to depolarize a nerve at the cathode (negative pole) than at the anode.[5] Of course, this is only meaningful when a direct or monophasic current is used.

Activity Questions:

1. Compare your findings with those of your partner. Do the motor points approximate those on the chart in Appendix B?

2. If you are using a unit where a polarity change is possible, try the following: Change the polarity from negative to positive. Move to an identified motor point and increase the intensity until a similar contraction is elicited. Was the required intensity greater than in your initial trial?

3. Is it possible to obtain a muscle contraction if not over a motor point? Why or why not?

Identification of Motor Points Worksheet

Name: ______________________ Date: ______________

Partner(s): ____

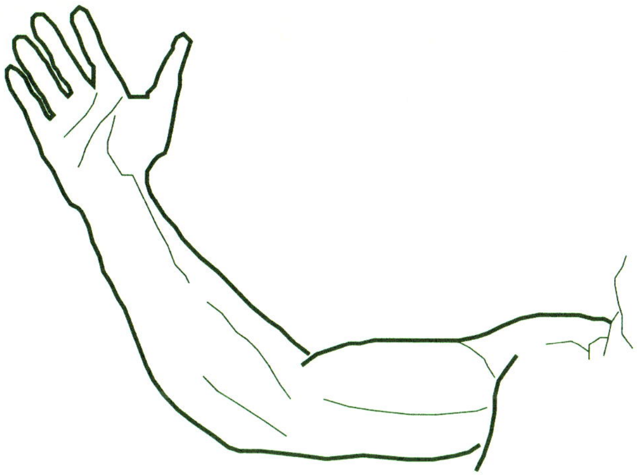

Arm - Anterior View

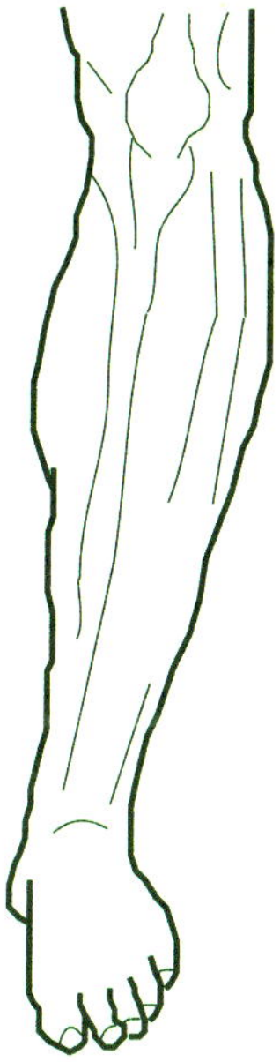

Leg - Anterior View

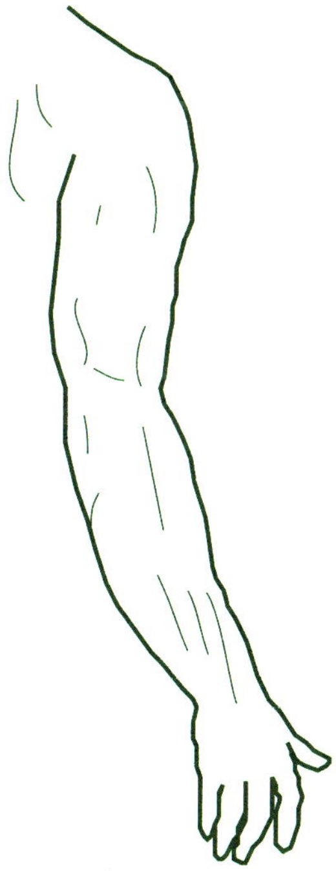

Arm - Posterior View

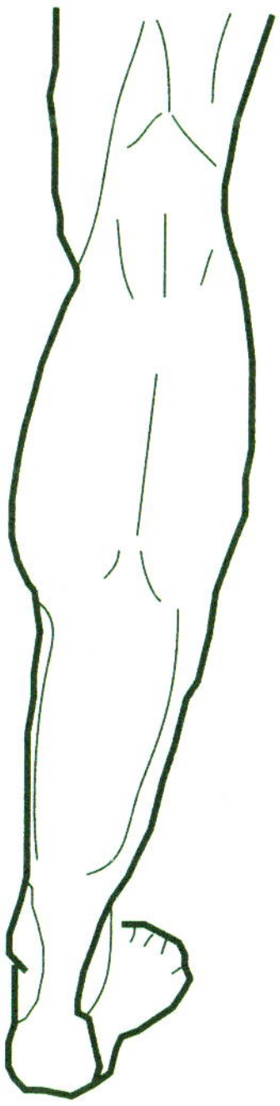

Leg - Posterior View

(Labeling key on reverse)

Labeling Key

Upper Extremity

1 Abductor pollicis
2 Extensor digiti minimi
3 Extensor indicis
4 Flexor carpi radialis
5 Flexor carpi ulnaris

6 Other: ______________________

7 Other: ______________________

8 Other: ______________________

9 Other: ______________________

10 Other: ______________________

Lower Extremity

A Abductor digiti minimi
B Extensor hallucis longus
C Peroneus longus
D Extensor digitorum brevis
E Tibialis anterior

F Other: ______________________

G Other: ______________________

H Other: ______________________

I Other: ______________________

J Other: ______________________

Class Activity 10

Manual Determination of Optimal Stimulation Sites

Objective: The student will manually determine superficial points on the skin having a decreased resistance to electrical stimulation, indicating primary stimulation points.

Materials Needed: Transcutaneous electrical nerve stimulation (TENS) unit or other electrical stimulator capable of a bipolar arrangement.

Procedures:

1. Using one channel of the TENS unit, set the stimulation parameters to the following values:

Pulse Duration:	20 μsec
Pulse Frequency:	120 pps
Modulation Parameters:	Off (constant output)

Note: Not all parameters will apply to each unit.

2. If required, apply conductive gel to each electrode. Attach one electrode to your dominant forearm and attach the other electrode to the subject's upper arm or lower leg, depending on the area being examined.

3. Apply a dab of conductive gel to the index finger of your dominant hand.

4. Touch the subject's extremity being examined (e.g., the forearm).

5. Slowly increase the output intensity of the TENS unit until a slight sensation is felt under your finger.

6. Slowly move your finger over the body area and note locations of increased sensation and whether or not a muscle contraction is associated with the particular point (Fig. 11). Label these locations on the chart provided.

7. Repeat this activity using another body part (e.g., the lower leg).

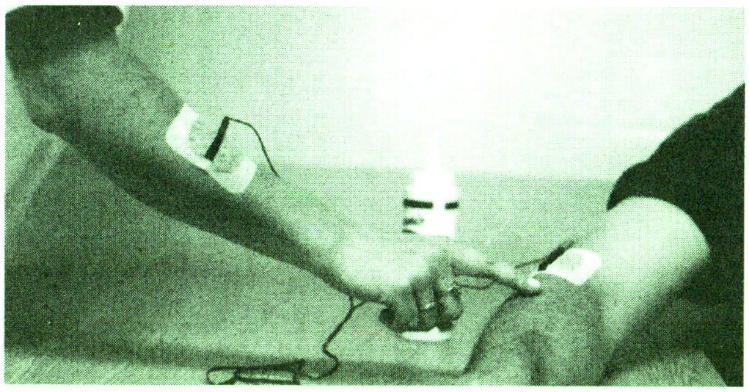

Figure 11. Setup for the manual determination of optimal stimulation sites.

Manual Determination of Optimal Stimulation Sites (Cont.)

Discussion:

In Class Activity 9, Identification of Motor Points, motor points are identified using a probe. Motor points, however, are not the only areas of decreased electrical resistance. Acupuncture points and trigger points also demonstrate diminished surface resistance to an electrical current. Ohm meters are often incorporated into many point stimulators to exactly locate these optimal stimulation site. In this activity, your finger is used as a quasi-ohm meter, and rather than a metered output to measure the amount of current flow, you are relying on your perception of the stimulus.

Activity Questions:

1. Review your results from Class Activity 9. Were you able to elicit contractions from approximately the same locations on the body?

2. What factor limited the maximal output intensity of the electrical stimulation device used in this activity?

3. Using the acupuncture chart located in Appendix C, attempt to locate as many points as possible along an upper or lower extremity meridian.

Manual Determination of Optimal Stimulation Sites Worksheet

Name: ______________________ Date: ______________

Partner(s): ______________________________________

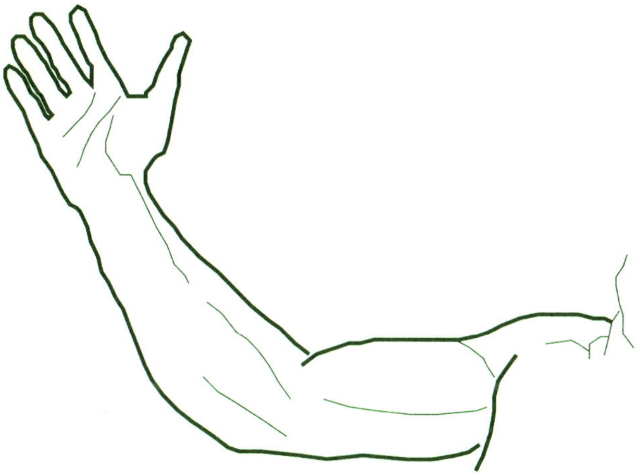

Arm - Anterior View

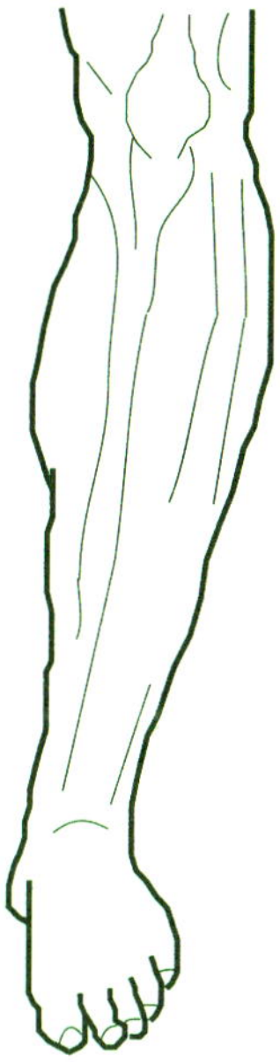

Leg - Anterior View

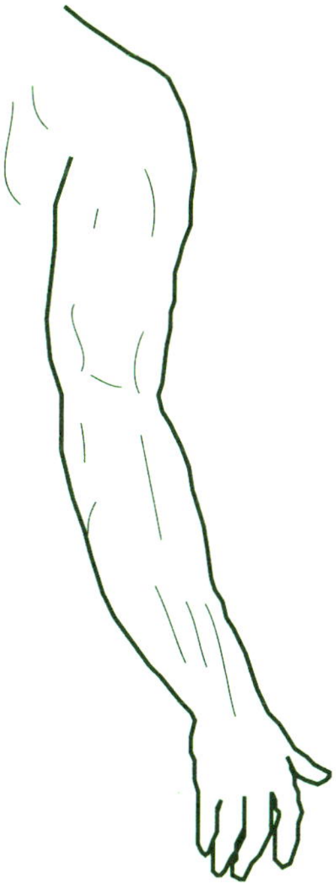

Arm - Posterior View

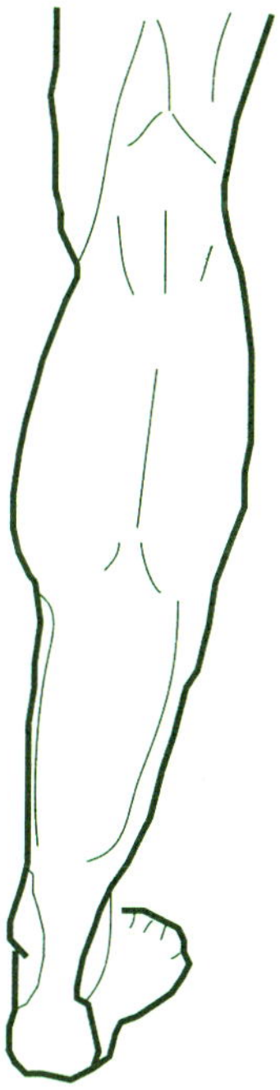

Leg - Posterior View

Labeling Key	
○ No Associated Muscle Contraction	● Associated Muscle Contraction

Class Activity 11

Strength of Electrically Elicited Muscle Contractions

Objective: The student will demonstrate the efficiency of various electrical stimulators, different electrode configurations, and varying electrical parameters in producing muscular tension in the quadriceps muscle group.

Materials Needed:
- High-volt pulsed stimulator
- Neuromuscular electrical stimulator
- Electromagnetic or hydraulic isokinetic dynamometer.

Measuring Electrically Induced Muscle Contractions:

As demonstrated in previous activities, an electrical current can be used to evoke a muscle contraction. Several factors influence the quality of these contractions, including the type of current, pulse duration, pulse frequency, output intensity, and electrode placement. The intensity of these contractions may be quantitatively measured using commercially available isokinetic units by comparing the force produced by an electrically induced involuntary isometric contraction (IIC) to that obtained by a maximal voluntary isometric contraction (MVIC).

After locking the limb in the position to be tested the subject performs a maximal isometric contraction of the quadriceps muscle, and the value is recorded. An electrical stimulation unit may then be configured to the extensor musculature and the force of the contraction is again measured (Fig. 12). Note that when the leg is hanging on the dynamometer, the output will read in negative numbers (e.g., -14 ft-lbs). This represents the force of gravity placing a force opposite that of the movement. Once the contraction, be it voluntary or involuntary, exceeds the force of gravity, these numbers will read as positive values.

The percentage of the MVIC obtained is determined by the formula: (IIC/MVIC) x 100.

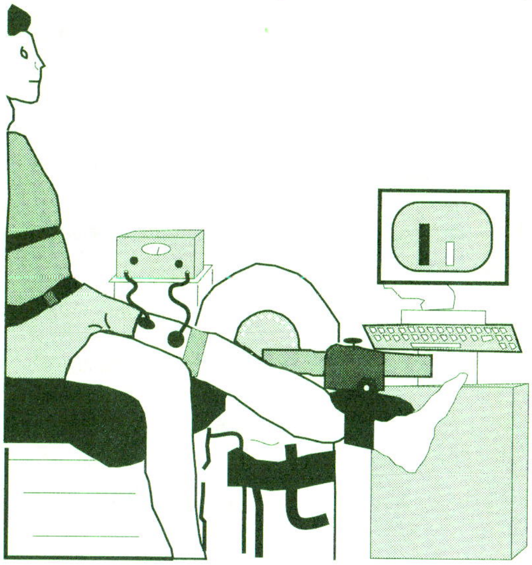

Figure 12. Configuration of isokinetic dynamometer and electrical stimulation unit.

Procedures:

1. Set up the dynamometer for isometric knee extension testing at approximately 70° of flexion according to the manufacturer's instructions.

2. Using the protocol specific to the dynamometer being used, determine the person's maximal voluntary isometric contraction force.

3. Using a high-volt pulsed stimulation unit and a monopolar configuration, attach the dispersive electrode on the leg opposite of that being tested. Place one active electrode over the proximal quadriceps and the other active electrode over the distal portion. The use of a motor point chart is recommended in identifying the optimal sites for electrode placement.

4. Configure the HVPS generator to the following parameters:

Pulse Duration:	Highest possible setting
Pulse Frequency:	30 pps
Pad Alternating Rate:	Continuous
Modulation Parameters:	Off
Current Ramp:	Fast (1 to 2 sec)
Duty Cycle:	50%

Note: Not all parameters will apply to each unit.

5. Increase the output intensity to the subject's tolerance. Note and record the maximal isometric tension produced by this method.

6. Reduce the intensity to zero and reconfigure the electrodes to a bipolar mode. This is easily done by disconnecting one of the active electrodes and inserting the lead from the dispersive electrode. The dispersive electrode is then removed from the body.

7. Increase the output intensity to the subject's tolerance. Note and record the maximal isometric tension produced by this method.

8. Remove the HVPS and apply the NMES in a bipolar configuration, again applying the electrodes over the proximal and distal quadriceps.

9. Configure the NMES to the following parameters:

Pulse Duration:	Highest possible setting
Pulse Frequency:	30 pps
Pulse Ramp:	Fast (1 to 2 sec)
Duty Cycle:	50%

Note: Not all parameters will apply to each unit.

10. Increase the output intensity to the subject's tolerance. Note and record the maximum isometric tension produced by this method.

Notes:

- Allow sufficient time for muscle recovery between bouts.
- This activity may be modified by altering the output parameters and electrode placement as well as changing the position of the lower extremity.
- It is not uncommon for the subject to experience muscle soreness following this activity.

Discussion:

An electrical current travels through the body by forming a sequence of parallel circuits, opting for the path of least resistance. Changing the configuration of the electrode placement alters the path of the current, although the area of greatest current density remains directly under the electrode(s) with the smallest surface area. The depth of the treatment effect corresponds to the proximity of the pads with the depth increasing as the space between the electrode increases.

The remaining variable to be considered is the electrodes' placement on or near motor points. As was seen in earlier exercises, stimulation of these finite points on the skin results in a stronger, more efficient contraction. If the current density over the muscle or muscle group is kept high, more motor points (and therefore motor units) will be recruited into the contraction. Increasing the output intensity by stimulating motor nerves in adjacent areas also has the same effect.

It was determined in the Selective Stimulation of Nerves (Class Activity 7) that sensory, motor, and pain nerves are sequentially recruited into the contraction. This concept should have been further reinforced by the fact that it was the subject's reporting of pain, rather than the limitations of the stimulating unit, that determined the maximal force that was produced, especially when units designed specifically for neuromuscular stimulation were used.

Activity Questions:

1. Based on the above discussion, would you expect a stronger contraction using a monopolar or bipolar pad arrangement? Did your results support this expectation?

2. For one of your trials using bipolar pad placement, change the frequency from 30 to 80 pps and compare the maximal involuntary isometric contraction strength. Is there any change? What explains this result?

3. Considering your results, which electrical stimulator would you use to obtain an optimal muscle contraction? Which pad placement?

4. Following a period of rest or using the opposite leg, plot the IIC using various duty cycles by altering the rest duration. What can be deduced from this activity regarding the implication of fatigue in electrically assisted muscle contractions?

Strength of Electrically Elicited Muscle Contractions Worksheet

Name: ______________________ Date: ______________

Partner(s): ____

Baseline Torque Production:

Maximal Voluntary Isometric Contraction	
Joint Angle	Peak Torque

Involuntary Torque Production:

Electrical Stimulator	Electrode Configuration	Pulse Duration	Pulses per Second	Duty Cycle	Max. Output Intensity	Joint Angle	Peak Torque	% MVIC

Class Activity 12

Effect of Cold Application in Reducing the Perception of Electrically Induced Pain

Objective: The student will determine if cold application before, or during electrical stimulation reduces the individual's perception of pain.

Materials Needed:
- Electrical stimulation unit with an adjustable pulse duration
- Crushed ice pack
- Ice massage cups.

Procedures:

1. Using a monopolar electrode configuration, attach the "dispersive" electrode on the subject's lower back or thigh and the "active" electrode to the anterior portion of the subject's forearm (this configuration is recommended for high volt pulsed units). If other stimulators are used, arrange the electrodes in a bipolar configuration with one electrode being placed on the distal portion of the subject's anterior forearm and the other on the proximal portion of the anterior forearm.

2. Set the stimulation parameters to the following values (it is recommended that the final parameters from Class Activity 7 also be used so that the results between these two exercises may be compared):

Pulse Duration:	160 μsec
Pulse Frequency:	30 pps
Pad Alternating Rate:	Continuous
Modulation Parameters:	Off (constant output)
Duty Cycle:	100%

Note: Not all parameters will be applicable to each unit.

3. Slowly increase the intensity until pain is experienced. Note and record the output intensity.

4. Reduce the intensity, remove the electrodes from the subject's forearm, and turn the generator off.

5. Apply a cold modality to the forearm until numbness is reported.

6. Reattach the electrodes and reapply the cold modality to the forearm.

7. Slowly increase the intensity until the subject reports pain. Note and record the output intensity.

8. Repeat this activity using multiple subjects or obtain the values obtained by other groups.

9. Statistical analysis, such as the t-test, may be used to determine if there is a significant difference between pain perception with and without concurrent cold application.

Discussion:

Cold application has been thought to decrease pain by decreasing the excitability of the pain-causing free nerve endings, stimulating of large diameter neurons, "closing the gate" as described by the gate control theory, and evoking descending inhibition through the central biasing mechanism. Cold modalities are frequently used for a temporary reduction of pain to enhance the subsequent treatment. For example, cold might be used before or during potentially painful active range of motion exercises in a technique known as cryokinetics. Additionally, as we have seen in Class Activity 11: Strength of Electrically Elicited Muscle Contractions, pain caused by the stimulating current determines the upper limits of torque production.

Research studies have been conducted to determine if cold application prior to electrical stimulation can increase the torque produced by an electrically evoked muscle contraction. One study using ice massage as the method for delivering cold found a significant increase in torque production compared to those receiving no such treatment.[6] A similar study using ice bags found no significant difference between the two groups.[7]

Questions:

1. Did the intensity at which pain was reported increase or decrease after the cold application?

2. Based on the results of this exercise, how would you explain the findings of the two research studies cited above?

Effect of Cold Application in Reducing the Perception of Electrically Induced Pain Worksheet

Name: ______________________ Date: ______________

Partner(s): ____

	Maximum Output Intensity		
Subject	No Cold Application	With Cold Application	Difference

Medical Galvanism

Objective: The student will see the difference in the migration of hydrogen and oxygen molecules between electrical modalities that use monophasic, biphasic, and direct currents.

Materials Needed:
- Monophasic current stimulator (e.g, HVPS)
- Biphasic stimulator (e.g., TENS)
- Galvanic stimulator (iontophoresor).
- Three beakers
- Distilled water

Description of Galvanism

Through an electromotive force, ions may be attracted to or repelled from electrical poles. Similar to magnetic poles, negatively charged ions are attracted to the positive pole, whereas positively charged ions are repelled from it, and vice versa for the negative pole (Fig. 13). Several treatment approaches, such as controlling the formation of edema, are based on this principle and the effectiveness is largely based on the type of current being used.

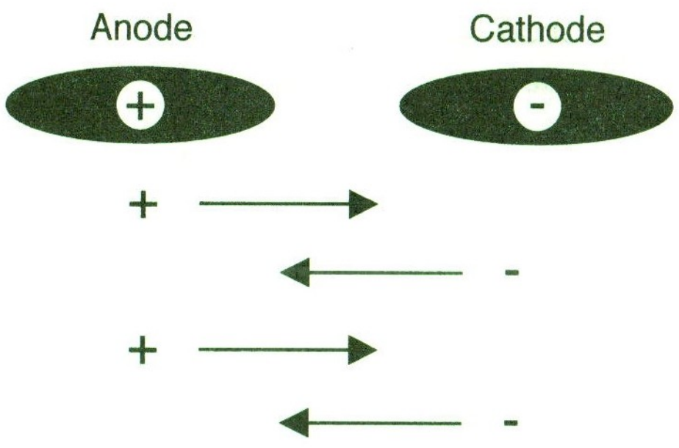

Figure 13. Movement of ions under the anode and the cathode.

Procedures:

1. Using distilled (degassed) water, fill three beakers.

2. In the three beakers, secure the bare electrode leads (from each of the three stimulators) approximately 2 to 3 inches apart from each other. Ensure that the leads are not touching the sides of the beaker or each other.

3. For those units delivering pulsed currents, set the output parameters to the highest possible number of pulses per second and the longest pulse duration. This parameter is not applicable to direct current (DC) generators. Where applicable, ensure that the output is constant (not modulated) and that the unit is operating at a 100% duty cycle.

4. Increase the intensity to the maximal possible output.

5. Allow the current to run for 10 minutes. **Do not disturb the units, beakers, or wires during the duration of this demonstration.**

6. At the end of the 10-minute period, note the number and size of the bubbles which are clinging to each electrode. The larger hydrogen should be attracted to the cathode (negative pole) and oxygen bubbles to the anode (positive pole).

Notes:

- Distilled water is available commercially, or tap water can be distilled by letting it sit uncovered for 24 hours.
- Prolonged use of stimulators using these parameters may result in damage to the equipment.

Discussion:

Your observations should have demonstrated that the largest number and largest sized bubbles were formed on the leads arising from the direct current generator. The size and number of bubbles on the leads from the monophasic current should be significantly less than those found on the direct current leads. No bubble formation should have been found on the leads emanating from the biphasic generator.

The direct current generator creates a continuous electromotive field between the anode and cathode. This allows for migration of hydrogen toward the cathode and oxygen to the anode. These lines of force between the polesof a monophasic generator are less distinct because of the interruption in the current flow. During the periods of noncurrent flow the ions are capable of freely drifting in any direction, ultimately reducing the net migration of the ions. The reason why there should be no bubble formation on the leads emanating from the biphasic generator is that no true anode or cathode pole exists, as each lead takes turns being the "positive" and "negative" pole. Any bubble formation is most likely the result of an extremely unbalanced pulse or artifact gasses in the water.

Class Exercise 1

Ohm's Law

Objective: The student will demonstrate an understanding of the relationship between voltage, amperage, resistance, and the power of an electrical circuit.

Description of Ohm's Law:

Ohm's law is a mathematical equation that describes a relationship where amperage (I) is directly proportional to voltage (V) and inversely proportional to resistance (R). Expressed as an equation, each variable can be calculated if the other two variables are known. To calculate:

Amperage	Voltage	Resistance:
$I = V/R$	$V = IR$	$R = V/I$

The total resistance to current flow is based on the type of electrical circuit involved. In a series circuit where the electrons have only one path which to travel, the total resistance is equal to the sum of all the resistors:

$$R_t = r_1 + r_2 + r_3 \ldots$$

In a parallel circuit, where electrons have multiple routes to travel, the total resistance is inversely proportional to the sum of the individual resistors:

$$R_t = 1/r_1 + 1/r_2 + 1/r_3$$

The power of a circuit is described in terms of watts and is calculated by the equation:

$$P = VI$$

Definition of Terms:

Amperage (I): The rate of electrical current flow as measured by the number of coulombs passing a single point in one second. One ampere is equal to the movement of one coulomb per second.

Coulomb (Q): Charge produced by 6.25×10^{18} electrons.

Ohm (Ω): Unit of electrical resistance. One ohm is the amount of resistance needed to develop 0.24 calories of heat when 1 ampere of current is applied for 1 second.

Voltage (V): The potential for electron flow to occur. One volt represents the amount of work required to move 1 coulomb of charge.

Watt (W): Unit of electrical power that describes the amount of work being performed in a unit of time.

Exercises

Respond to the following questions using the schematics provided below:

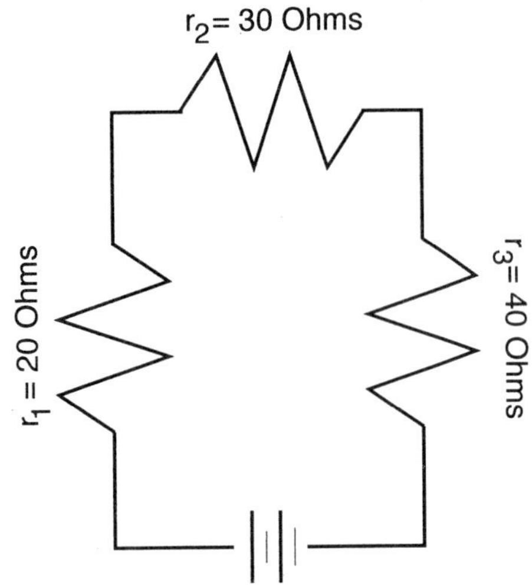

Series Circuit

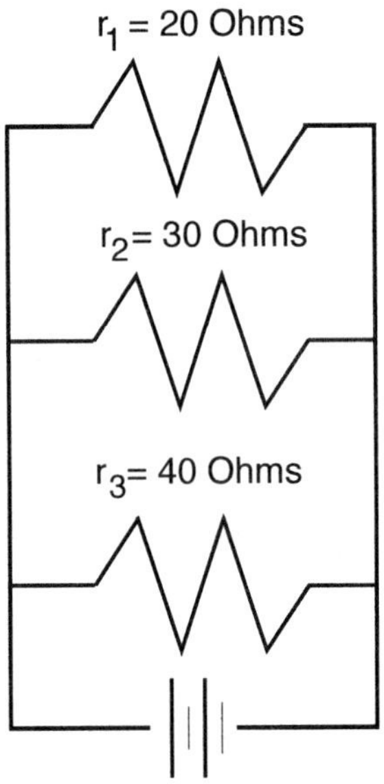

Parallel Circuit

1. What is the total resistance in the series circuit? The parallel circuit?

2. Using the resistance value obtained in question 1, what would be the amperage of each circuit if each is operating at 120 volts?

3. What would the amperage for each of the two circuits be if the voltage were increased to 200 volts?

4. Using the parameters from question 2, what would the wattage be for each circuit type?

5. Calculate the voltage across each resistor in the series circuit assuming the circuit is operating at 10 amperes.

6. Calculate the amperage across each resistor in the parallel circuit assuming it is operating at 100 volts and 10 amperes.

7. Calculate the total resistance in the parallel circuit after adding two additional resistors of 30 ohms each.

8. Using the total resistance value obtained from question 7, calculate the amperage if the circuit is operating at 120 volts.

9. Compare your answers to questions 8 and 2 for the amperage of the parallel circuit. After adding resistance, did the amperage increase or decrease? Why?

Class Exercise 2

Pulse Characteristics

Objective: The student will demonstrate knowledge of the characteristics associated with therapeutic currents.

Electrical Stimulating Currents:

Direct Current: The uninterrupted unidirectional flow of electrons.

Alternating Current: The uninterrupted bidirectional flow of electrons.

Pulsed Current: The flow of electrons interrupted by discrete periods of noncurrent flow.

Monophasic Current: A unidirectional pulsed current.

Biphasic Current: A pulsed current possessing two phases, each which occurs on opposite sides of the baseline.

Definition of Pulse Characteristics:

Amplitude: The maximal distance that a pulse rises above or below the baseline.

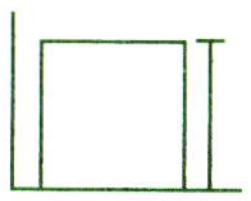

Interpulse Interval: The period of time between pulses during which there is no current flow.

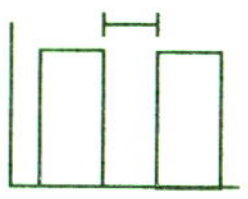

Intrapulse Interval: The period of time within a single pulse during which there is no current flow. The duration of the intrapulse interval cannot exceed the duration of the interpulse interval.

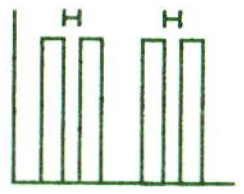

Peak-to-Peak Amplitude: The absolute value measured from the maximal rise on the positive side of the baseline to the peak on the negative side.

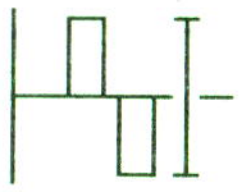

Pulse Duration: The period of time a pulse remains above or below the baseline, normally measured in microseconds.

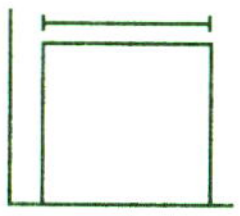

Pulse Frequency: With pulsed currents this figure represents the number of pulses per second (pps); alternating currents are measured by the number of cycles per second (cps or hertz).

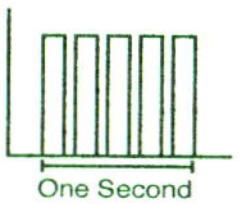

Pulse Period: The period of time between the initiation of one pulse to the initiation of the subsequent pulse.

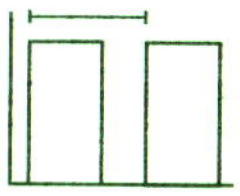

Exercises:

1. Label each of the following current types, indicating the specified parameter. If a particular parameter is not applicable to a particular current, leave it blank.

A. Identify the amplitude for each of the following currents:

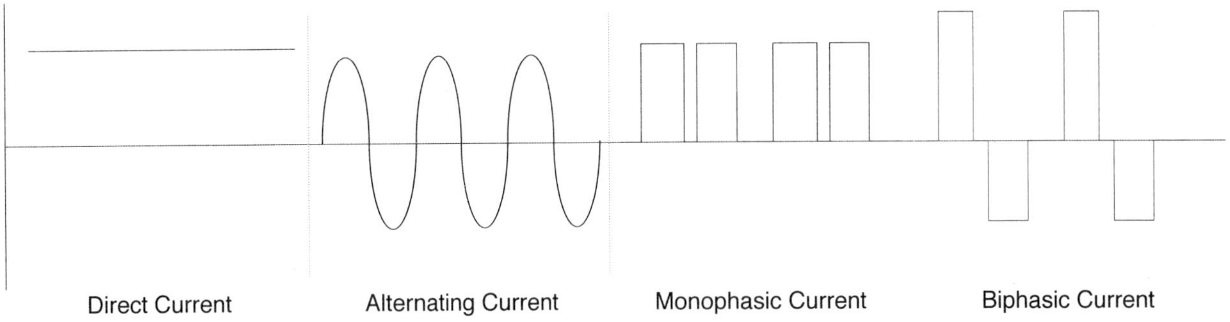

B. Identify the peak-to-peak value for each of the following currents:

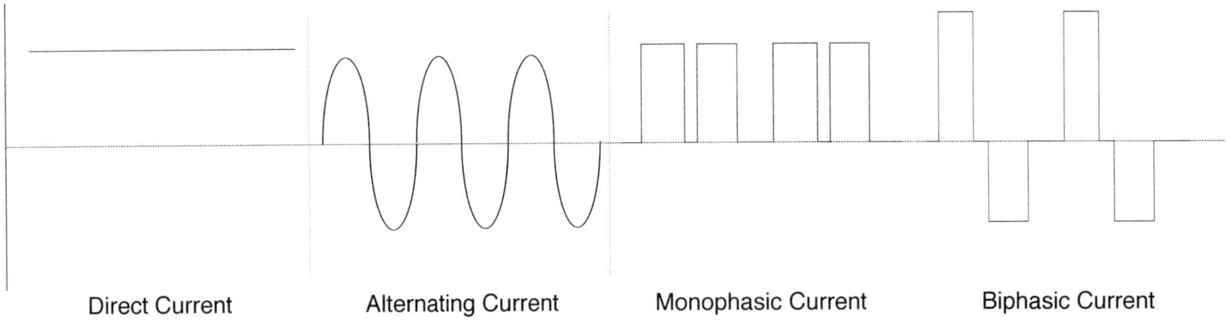

C. Identify the pulse duration for each of the following currents:

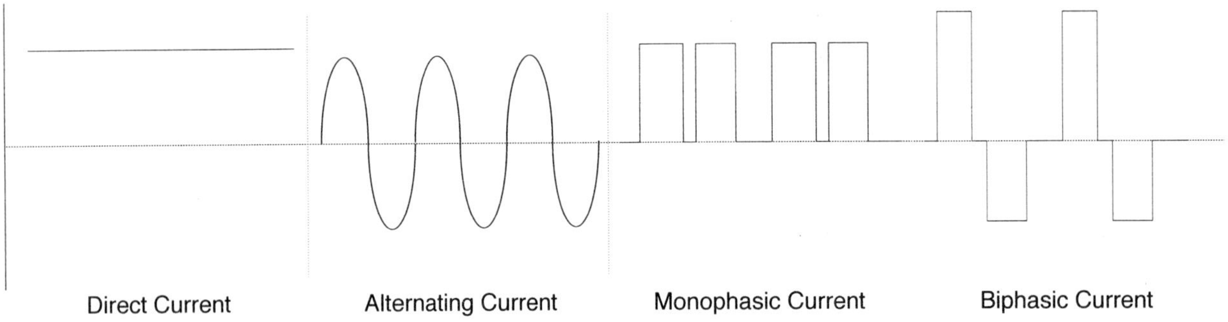

D. Identify the pulse period for each of the following currents:

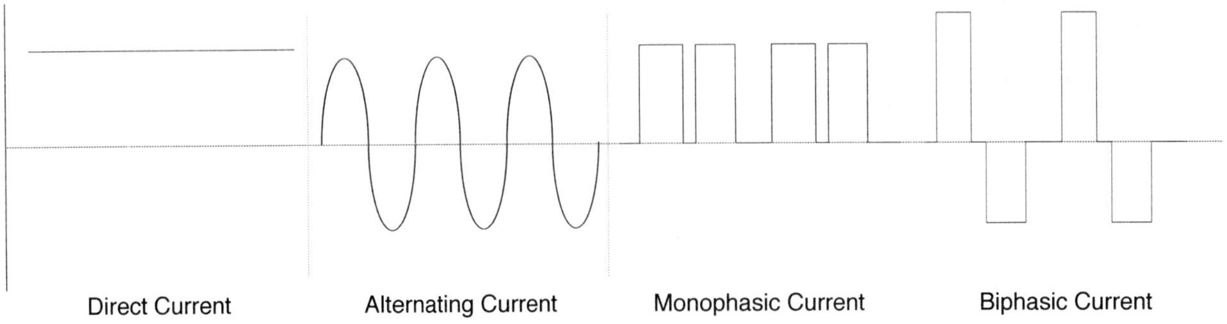

E. Identify the interpulse interval for each of the following currents:

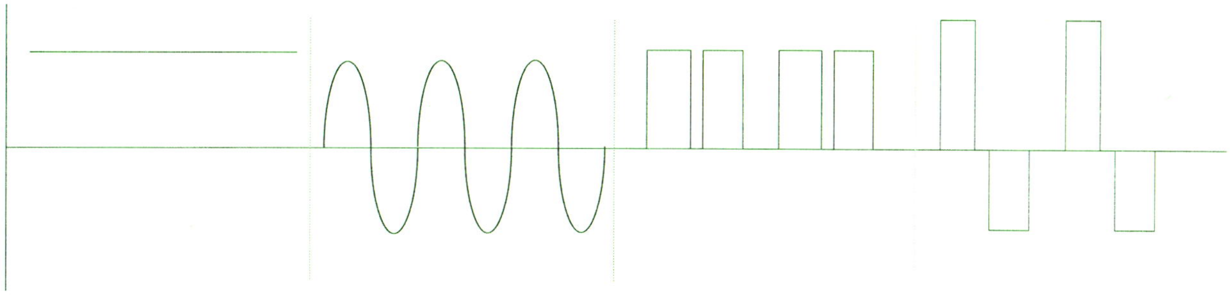

Direct Current | Alternating Current | Monophasic Current | Biphasic Current

F. Identify the intrapulse interval for each of the following currents:

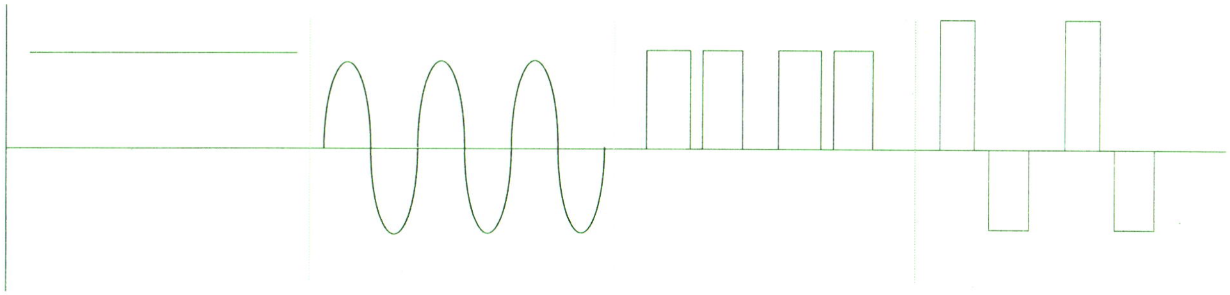

Direct Current | Alternating Current | Monophasic Current | Biphasic Current

2. Calculate the total amount of time electrons are actually moving during a 1-minute period in a pulsed current having a pulse duration of 140 μsec and a frequency of 125 pps.

3. The amount of energy delivered to the tissue is represented by the area within a pulse. What two variables can we manipulate to increase or decrease this energy?

Class Activity 14

Coupling Ability of Various Ultrasound Media

Objective: The student will determine the relative ability of various media to transmit ultrasonic energy.

Materials Needed:
- Ultrasound unit
- Athletic tape or similar
- Various ultrasound transmission media (e.g., commercial transmission gels, hydrocortisone mixtures, petroleum jelly)

Procedures:

1. Configure the ultrasound unit to continuous output and, if adjustable, the output meter to total watts (W).
2. Using athletic tape (or something similar), form a well around the ultrasound head (Fig. 14).
3. Fill the well with water.
4. Turn the unit on and slowly increase the intensity until a steady movement (bubbling or agitation) of the water is seen.
5. Record the output intensity in total watts and reset the unit.
6. For ease of application, remove the tape and completely cover the ultrasound head with an even layer of coupling gel. Re-form the well with tape and fill with water. Repeat steps 4 and 5.
7. Using other media, repeat step 6.
8. If available, repeat this exercise using a sound head of a different size.

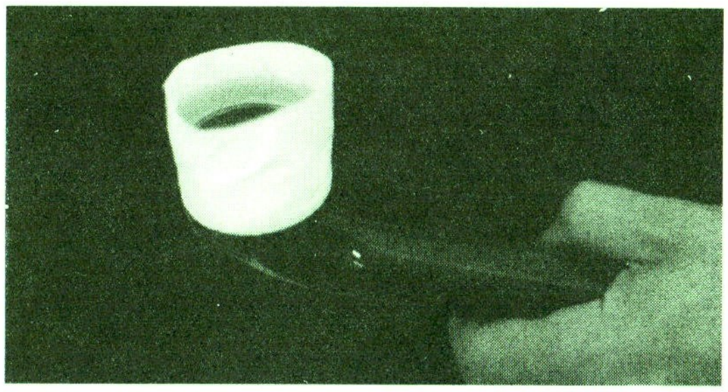

Figure 14. Taping the ultrasound head to form a well.

Notes:

- If available, a commercial ultrasound output meter (such as those used for calibrating the instrument) may be used.
- Caution must be practiced when using older ultrasound generators that do not have an automatic shut-off feature built in. Continually running the sound head when the energy is not being transmitted (such as holding the transducer in the air and turning up the intensity) may seriously damage the crystal.

Discussion:

Because ultrasonic energy cannot be transmitted through the air, an adequate coupling medium must be used to ensure that the sound waves are being transmitted to the tissues. All commercially available approved coupling gels meet this task. However, many times clinicians will substitute these with other forms of media, especially during phonophoresis treatments.

Many of the different media with which hydrocortisone is mixed are totally incapable of transmitting ultrasonic energy. Likewise, many other phonophoresis media, such as Theragesic™ or Aspercreme™ have little or no ability to transmit ultrasound. Generally speaking, thick, white creams (such as hand/skin creams) are poor conductors, whereas gel-mixed agents serve as good conductors.[7]

Activity Questions:

1. Which medium served as the best conductor of ultrasonic energy? Why do you think this is?

2. Which medium appeared to be the least effective conductor of ultrasonic energy? Why do you think this is?

3. Many of the media customarily used as bases for phonophoresis are not good conductors of ultrasonic energy, yet many individuals still report benefits from the treatment. Why do you think this occurs?

Coupling Ability of Various Ultrasound Media Worksheet

Name: ______________________ Date: ______________

Partner(s): ______________________________________

ERA of sound head:

Coupling Medium	Watts Needed to Cause "Bubbles"

ERA of sound head:

Coupling Medium	Watts Needed to Cause "Bubbles"

Ultrasound Output Worksheet

Objective: The student will display a mastery of the concepts associated with therapeutic ultrasound.

Definition of Terms:

Beam Nonuniformity Ratio (BNR): The ratio between the spatial peak intensity to the average output as reported on unit's meter.

Duty Cycle: The ratio between the ultrasound's pulse length and pulse interval when ultrasound is being delivered in the pulsed mode.

Effective Radiating Area (ERA): The area of the ultrasound head that produces mechanical waves, normally measured in square centimeters (cm^2).

Near Field: The portion of the ultrasound beam that is used for therapeutic purposes.

Spatial Average Intensity (SAI): The amount of ultrasound energy passing through the ultrasound head, expressed in watts per square centimeter (W/cm^2).

Spatial Peak Intensity (SPI): The maximum output (power) produced within an ultrasound beam.

Temporal Average Intensity (TAI): The power of ultrasonic output over a period of time. This measure is only meaningful with pulsed ultrasound.

Ultrasound: Mechanical sound waves occurring at frequency above the range of human hearing (> 20,000 Hz). Therapeutic ultrasound ranges between 1 and 3 MHz.

Exercises

1. Using an ultrasound unit having a 4:1 BNR, the metered output indicates that an average of 4 watts of power is being delivered to the tissues. What is the peak intensity being delivered to the tissues in this treatment?

2. The spatial average intensity of an ultrasound treatment is dependent on the effective radiating area of the sound head. Calculate the output, in watts per square centimeter, for an ultrasound beam at an intensity of 5 watts for the following sound heads, each having a different ERA:

ERA	W/cm^2
10 cm^2	
8 cm^2	
5 cm^2	
3 cm^2	
1 cm^2	

3. Using the parameters cited below, calculate the percent duty cycle and the temporal average intensity assuming that the metered output displays 4 W/cm^2:

Pulse Duration (sec)	Pulse Interval (sec)	% Duty Cycle	Temporal Average Intensity
10	10		
20	40		
10	50		
25	50		

Class Activity 15

Strength of Biofeedback-Augmented Muscle Contractions

Objective: The student will determine the effectiveness of visual and/or auditory biofeedback, or both, in increasing voluntary isometric contraction of the quadriceps muscle group.

Materials Needed:
- Single-channel biofeedback unit
- Electromagnetic or hydraulic isokinetic device

Procedures:

1. See Class Activity 11, Strength of Electrically Elicited Muscle Contractions, for a description of measuring the strength of muscle contractions.
2. Set up the dynamometer for isometric knee extension testing at approximately 15° of flexion according to the manufacturer's instructions.
3. Using the protocol specific to the dynamometer being used, determine the subject's maximal voluntary isometric contraction (MVIC) force. Record this value on the chart provided.
4. Using the recommended coupling medium, attach the three biofeedback electrodes to the oblique fibers of the vastus medialis, making sure that the "active" electrodes are directly over the muscle belly. (The "reference" electrode is commonly black or red and is often placed to form a triangle with the two active electrodes.)
5. Find the threshold electromyographic (EMG) level that the subject can achieve only through near-maximal isometric contraction.
6. Select one of three biofeedback parameters: (a) metered feedback only, (b) audio feedback only, or (c) both metered and audio feedback.
7. Measure the MVIC produced in conjunction with each of the three feedback methods described in number 6 above.

Notes:

- If a biofeedback unit is not available, perform this exercise in two bouts, one in which the subject cannot see the dynamometer's output display and one in which the subject can see the display.
- Muscle soreness may be experienced following the completion of this activity.

Discussion:

While unable to directly measure the force of a muscle contraction, (EMG) biofeedback can assess the electrical correlate to that contraction and provide this information to the user in the form of visual and/or auditory feedback. EMG biofeedback units typically have three electrodes, with two used to gather information from the muscle and the third acts as a reference electrode, filtering unwanted information.

Strength of Biofeedback-Augmented Muscle Contractions (Cont.)

Biofeedback is ideally used early in the rehabilitation process to re-establish neurological pathways lost because of immobilization or nerve damage. Even though healthy muscle is used in this exercise, the concept of monitoring electrical activity in the muscle is the same. If we were attempting to re-educated unhealthy or unused muscle, the procedures and principles would remain the same, and only a lower threshold would be used.

Activity Questions:

1. Under which condition, if any, was the baseline MVIC exceeded?

2. Explain the similarities and differences between biofeedback and other feedback types (e.g., touching the muscle, yelling encouragement).

Strength of Biofeedback-Augmented Muscle Contractions Worksheet

Name: ______________________ Date: ______________

Partner(s): ____

Subject	Maximum Voluntary Contraction Force Produced			
	No Feedback (%)	Visual Feedback (%)	Audio Feedback (%)	Both (%)

Class Activity 16

Educating Muscle with Biofeedback

Objective: The student will understand the principles and effects of educating muscle through electromyographic (EMG) biofeedback by eliciting a voluntary unilateral eyebrow raise.

Materials Needed:
- EMG biofeedback
- Mirror

Procedures:

1. Place the electrodes over the occipitofrontalis muscle located above one of the eyebrows (Fig. 15).
2. Adjust the biofeedback threshold to the lowest sensitivity level that does not produce feedback of electrical activity at rest.
3. Position the mirror (or provide verbal feedback) so that the subject will be aware of a unilateral rather than a bilateral raising of the eyebrow.
4. Continue to decrease the sensitivity of the biofeedback unit as the subject's muscle becomes educated to the contraction.
5. Once the subject learns how to accomplish this task, remove the electrodes and have the subject attempt to raise an eyebrow without the assistance of biofeedback.

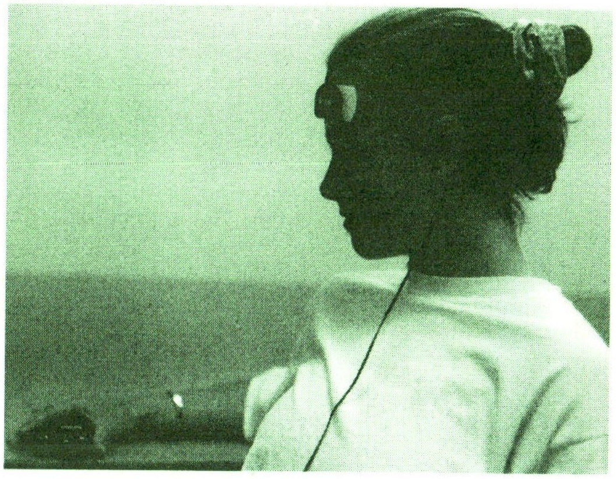

Figure 15. Electrode placement for determining electrical activity in the occipitofrontalis muscle.

Note:

- If the subject can already perform a unilateral eyebrow raise, attempt to elicit a contraction from another rarely used muscle such as the auricularis superior, which raises the ear superiorly and posteriorly.

Discussion:

In this activity we are substituting a healthy muscle that is rarely used for a damaged muscle to illustrate how neural pathways can be established. The biofeedback unit is being used as a learning tool to increase the subject's awareness and subsequently assist in the neural development of the pathways necessary to contract a muscle. Because the final goal of EMG biofeedback is unassisted voluntary contraction, the final phase of each treatment session should conclude with an exercise bout without the assistance of feedback.

Activity Questions:

1. During the early stages of this exercise it is not uncommon for both eyebrows to rise. To what neurophysiological principle do you attribute this tendency?

2. Using these principles, describe how you would employ EMG biofeedback to promote muscular relaxation.

Class Activity 17

Supine vs. Sitting Cervical Traction

Objective: To determine the effects of gravity on the force needed for cervical traction.

Materials Needed:
- Cervical traction unit
- 20-pound weight and an assortment of other free weights

Procedures:

1. Attach the rope from the traction unit to the 20-pound weight, allowing the weight to rest freely from the unit.
2. If a mechanical traction unit is being used, turn it on. If a pulley system is being used, begin to add weight in measurable increments (Fig. 16).
3. Gradually increase the tension until the weight begins to rise. Record the tension at the point where the weight is first lifted from the table.
4. Reposition the traction unit so that the weight will be pulled across the table (see Fig. 16). Gradually increase the tension until the weight begins to slide. Record this value on the chart provided.
5. Repeat steps 1 through 5 using different weights.

Note:

- If a commercial traction unit is not available, this activity can be performed using a rope and free weights in 1- and 2-pound increments.

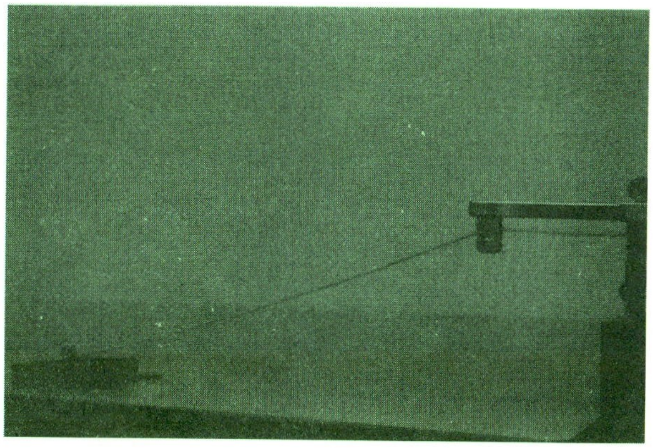

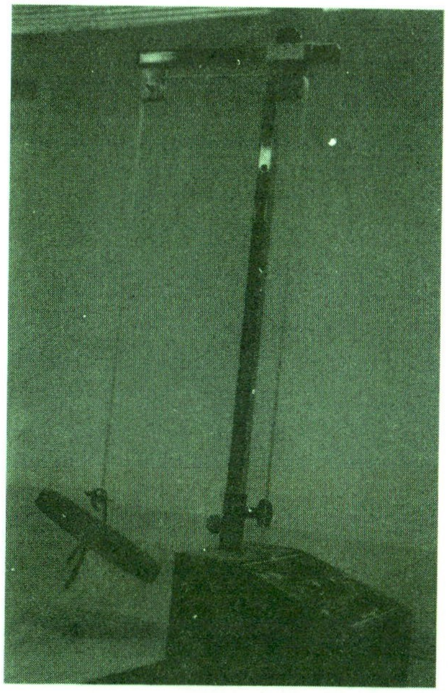

Figure 16. Set up of a mechanical cervical traction unit for supine (left) vs. sitting (right) cervical traction.

Discussion:

In this activity, the 20-pound weight approximates the weight of the human head. The effects of gravity become apparent in the increased load necessary to lift rather than slide the weight. The therapeutic effects of cervical traction will not be realized until the forces of gravity are overcome. For this reason, cervical traction applied in the supine position is preferred over cervical traction in the sitting position. The benefit of muscle relaxation is also added when the person is supine.

Activity Questions:

1. What was the difference between the amount of tension required to raise the weight vertically compared to the amount of tension required to slide the weight across the table? Did this percentage remain constant when other weights were used?

2. What other factors account for the amount of tension required to slide the weight across the table?

Supine vs. Sitting Cervical Traction Worksheet

Name: ______________________ Date: ______________

Partner(s): ____

	Force Required			% of Dummy Weight		
Weight	Vertical	Horizontal		Vertical	Horizontal	% Difference
20 lbs.						

Case Studies

The following case studies are presented to test your clinical decision making and knowledge of the clinical parameters of therapeutic modalities in the development of treatment plans. Depending on your background and the directions from your instructor, you may also incorporate therapeutic exercise into your treatment plan.

Unless otherwise directed, assume that you have all necessary equipment at your disposal. Assume that the patients described in these case studies are healthy unless stated in the text or by your instructor. These case studies may be modified by repeating them with only a limited number of modalities or by ascribing certain disease states to the individual.

A listing of patient problems that should be addressed during the treatment and rehabilitation of these conditions is provided in Appendix G.

Case Study 1

A 21 year old (y/o) wrestler sustained a left quadriceps contusion 4 days ago when he was struck by an opponent's knee.

Subjective Findings:

- patient complains of pain, weakness, and stiffness in the left quadriceps
- patient reports reduction of symptoms following ice application

Objective Findings:

- painful gait: rating 5/10
- mild localized swelling with no discoloration
- injured area is point tender with no noticeable temperature increase
- pain with active contraction of the left quadriceps
- passive range of motion (PROM): 0° to 90°
- active range of motion (AROM): 10° to 90°

Based on the above information, develop a problem list and detail a treatment plan for this patient.

Case Study 2

A 25 y/o soccer player suffered an inversion ankle sprain of her right ankle 24 hours ago. Her chief complaint is an inability to fully bear weight without pain.

Subjective Findings:

- patient complains of pain with weight bearing and constant aching in the right ankle
- prior history of similar injuries to the right ankle

Objective Findings:

- slight limp from lack of push-off during gait
- mild swelling located in the lateral ankle and foot
- point tenderness over anterior talofibular ligament; mild warmth
- full AROM; pain 7/10 with active movement
- negative anterior drawer test
- manual muscle test findings:

  3+/5 evertors
  4/5 invertors
  4/5 dorsiflexors
  3/5 plantarflexors

Based on the above information, develop a problem list and detail a treatment plan for this patient. How would your treatment differ if significant edema was present?

Case Study 3

A 43 y/o patient has had a traumatic adhesive capsulitis in her left shoulder for the past 5 months. Symptoms have decreased since the initiation of therapeutic exercise and mobilization 2 weeks ago, but abduction and external rotation of the humerus are still limited.

Subjective Findings:

- pain with daily activities: reports 60% function
- complains of a diffuse and intermittent aching sensation, especially around the insertion of the deltoid muscle
- reports that joint mobilization and home stretching program have improved range of motion

Objective Findings:

- pain rating 4/10
- no point tenderness
- left shoulder AROM:

    abduction: 0° to 80°
    flexion: 0° to 100°
    external rotation: 0° to 15°
    internal rotation: 0° to 20°

- springy end-feels in all directions; reduced capsular glide, especially anteriorly and inferiorly
- scapular substitution pattern with active motion

Based on the above information, develop a problem list and detail a treatment plan for this patient. How should the patient be positioned to get optimal treatment effects?

Case Study 4

A 17 y/o patient has been removed from a long leg cast after 4 weeks of immobilization for a grade III medial collateral ligament (MCL) sprain. He has been given clearance to perform strengthening exercises as tolerated and has no restrictions. He is having difficulty generating a strong quadriceps contraction.

Subjective Findings:

- patient injured left knee while skiing; had immediate dysfunction and was unable to walk
- MRI revealed a complete MCL disruption with small, peripheral medial meniscus tear
- patient has been immobilized in 25° of flexion for 4 weeks
- patient now wearing hinged brace with its ROM adjusted to tolerance
- patient weight bearing as tolerated with crutches until normal gait returns

Objective Findings:

- joint line tenderness at MCL
- pain rating 3/10
- minimal effusion; slight thickening at suprapatellar pouch
- marked quadriceps atrophy (5 cm girth difference, 10 cm above medial joint line)
- AROM: 12° to 95°
- PROM: 5° to 105°

Based on the above information, develop a problem list and detail a treatment plan for this patient. What home program would you give this patient?

Case Study 5

A swimmer complains of recurrent right shoulder pain which has increased over the last 2 weeks. She describes the pain as a vague, aching sensation that somewhat resolves with ice and rest. Heat application prior to swimming irritates the condition. Her chief complaint is pain late in the evening and at night despite the use of an ice pack several times a day. She is concerned about her participation in the upcoming Olympic trials.

Subjective Findings:

- patient complains of pain in right shoulder, especially during warm-up and after practice
- ice and exercises have decreased symptoms over the past 2 weeks

Objective Findings:

- reported pain 8/10; pain usually decreases after several minutes of swimming but is reported at 5/10 with activity
- pain on palpation at the posterior aspect of the glenohumeral joint
- full AROM and PROM of the upper extremity and cervical spine
- generalized laxity at glenohumeral joint, especially with anterior shear

Based on the above information, develop a problem list and detail a treatment plan for this patient.

Case Study 6

A 73 y/o retired carpenter had a total knee replacement 15 days ago. He has been given clearance for rehabilitation. The surgeon's only restriction is to limit weight-bearing to 50% for the next 4 weeks. The patient's chief complaint is stiffness.

Subjective Findings:

- patient has had degenerative joint dysfunction for past 25 years
- past medical history significant for controlled hypertension and mild cardiovascular disease
- patient is ambulatory and partial weight bearing with crutches

Objective Findings:

- incision closed and healing well
- reported pain 2/10
- moderate effusion
- decreased patellar mobility
- anesthetic area around incision
- AROM: 18° to 93°
- PROM: 4° to 97°

Based on the above information, develop a problem list and detail a treatment plan for this patient. When would ultrasound be incorporated in the program to augment ROM exercises?

Two weeks later, the patient continues to have a 15° active extension lag. The effusion has decreased. How would you modify your treatment plan to meet this patient's current needs?

Case Study 7

A 37 y/o mother of 3 small children is 6 weeks status post right ankle bimalleolar fracture treated with an open reduction and internal fixation. She has just returned from the physician's visit where the short leg cast was removed. Her primary goal is independent daily activities, including child care.

Subjective Findings:

- patient tripped on stairs and fractured right ankle 6 weeks ago
- patient is full weight bearing
- patient complains of stiffness, aching, and swelling

Objective Findings:

- mild pain with gait; right foot turns out to accommodate for decreased ROM
- incisions well healed; skin dry and flaky; no palpable warmth
- pitting edema on dorsum of foot
- AROM: 5° to 22° plantarflexion
- PROM: 0° to 28° plantarflexion

Based on the above information, develop a problem list and detail a treatment plan for this patient. Her insurance will only pay for 2 visits per week for 3 weeks.

Case Study 8

A 27 y/o male sustained a below knee amputation to his left leg following a motorcycle accident. The surgery was 10 weeks ago, and he is now ready to begin gait-training with a prosthesis. His chief complaint is stiffness in his knee.

Subjective Findings:

- patient has minimal complaints of pain in residual limb or knee
- patient has been sleeping with a pillow under knee for comfort

Objective Findings:

- well healed incision
- no palpable tenderness at the knee or residual limb
- knee AROM: 15° to 130°
- hamstrings markedly tight

Based on the above information, develop a problem list and detail a treatment plan for this patient.

Appendix A

Methods to Monitor Skin Surface Temperature

The ideal method to monitor the surface temperature of the skin during and after the application of thermal modalities is with an electronic sensor specifically designed for this purpose. These devices have a special sensor in their tips which allows them to measure temperature rapidly and accurately. Their output is displayed with either an analog meter or a more accurate digital readout.

These meters are not "run-of-the-day" items and may not be found in many educational settings. The following devices have been used in lieu of these more "high-tech" devices:

Electronic Outdoor Thermometer

Digital outdoor thermometers (those possessing wired leads) may be used to accurately measure changes in skin temperature. We recommend placing the sensor on the skin and then covering it with a 2- by 3-inch piece of Neoprene™ material (cut from an old knee sleeve) during the temperature reading (Fig. 17). Experimentation is needed with individual units to determine the amount of time required to fully read the temperature change. Advantages of this type of unit include accuracy by way of a digital readout, and some units have memories in which temperature readings may be stored. Radio Shack® has a line of electronic thermometers, with costs ranging from $15 to $30.

Household Thermometers

Standard mercury thermometers having a temperature range between 40°F and 130°F will suffice for the exercises in this workbook. The only requirement is that the bulb end of the thermometer must be exposed to allow contact with the subject's skin. As with the electronic outdoor thermometer, we recommend covering the bulb and skin with a 2- by 3-inch piece of Neoprene™ material during the temperature reading. For maximal accuracy, the bulb and lower stem of the thermometer must remain in contact with the subject's skin during the reading.

General Instructions

With either instrument, remove the Neoprene™ covering when temperatures are not being taken so that the cooling or warming process is not incorrectly influenced.

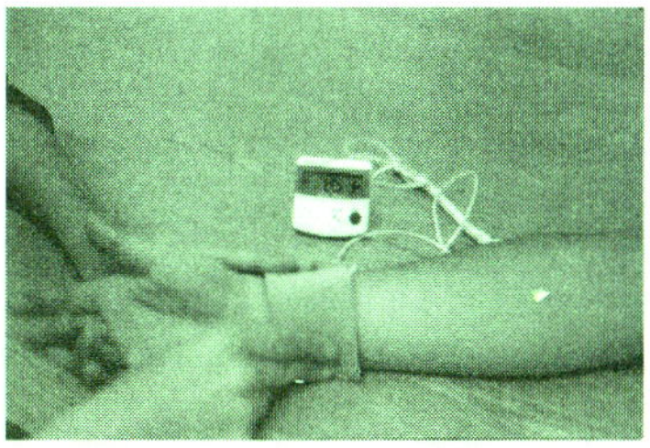

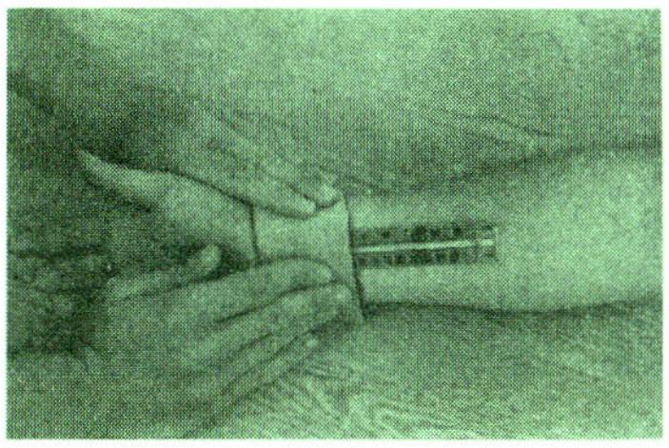

Figure 17. Set up for the use of an electronic thermometer (left) and a mercury-based outdoor thermometer.

Motor Point Chart

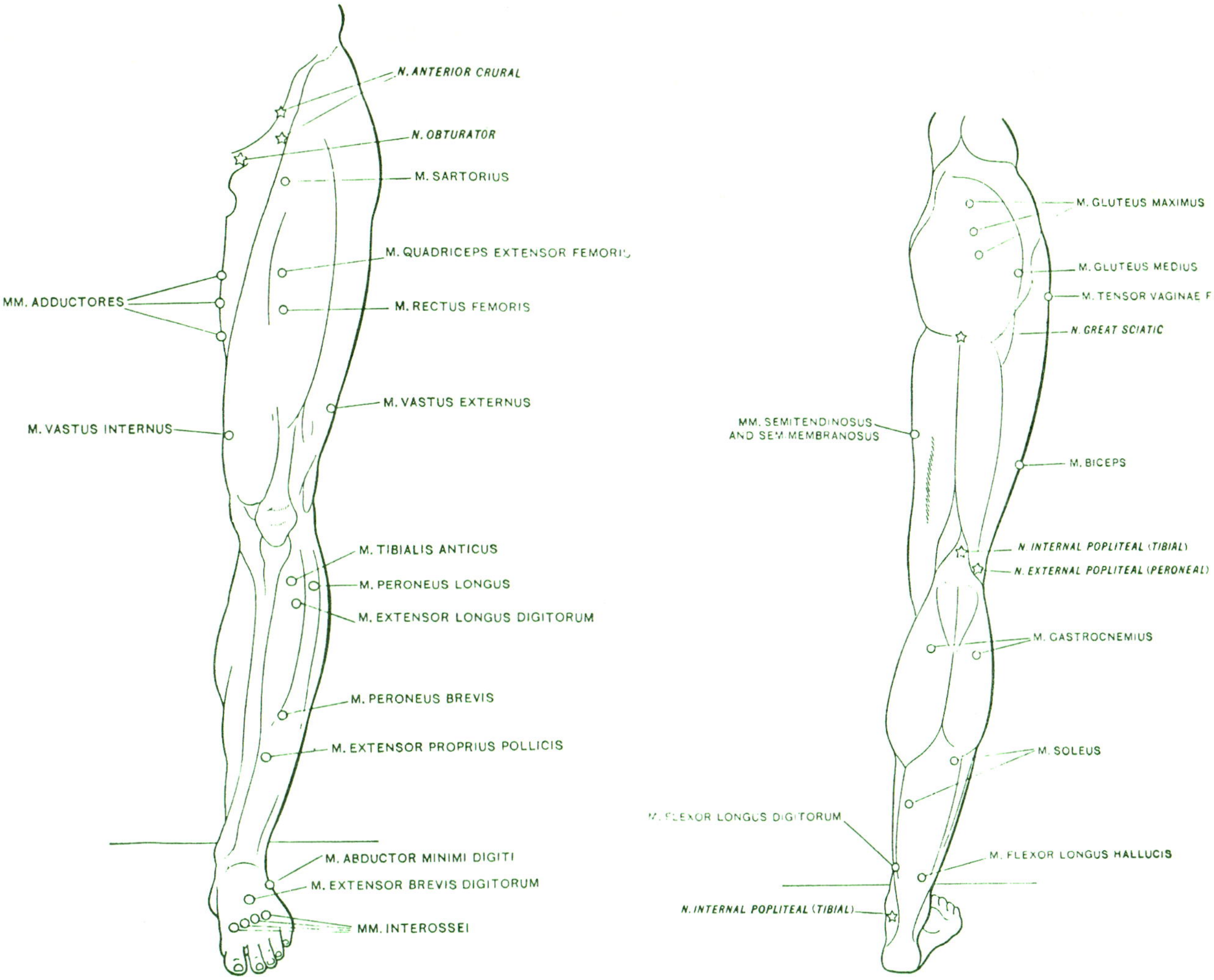

M = Muscle
N = Nerves

From Mettler Electronics® Corporation, Anaheim, California, with permission.

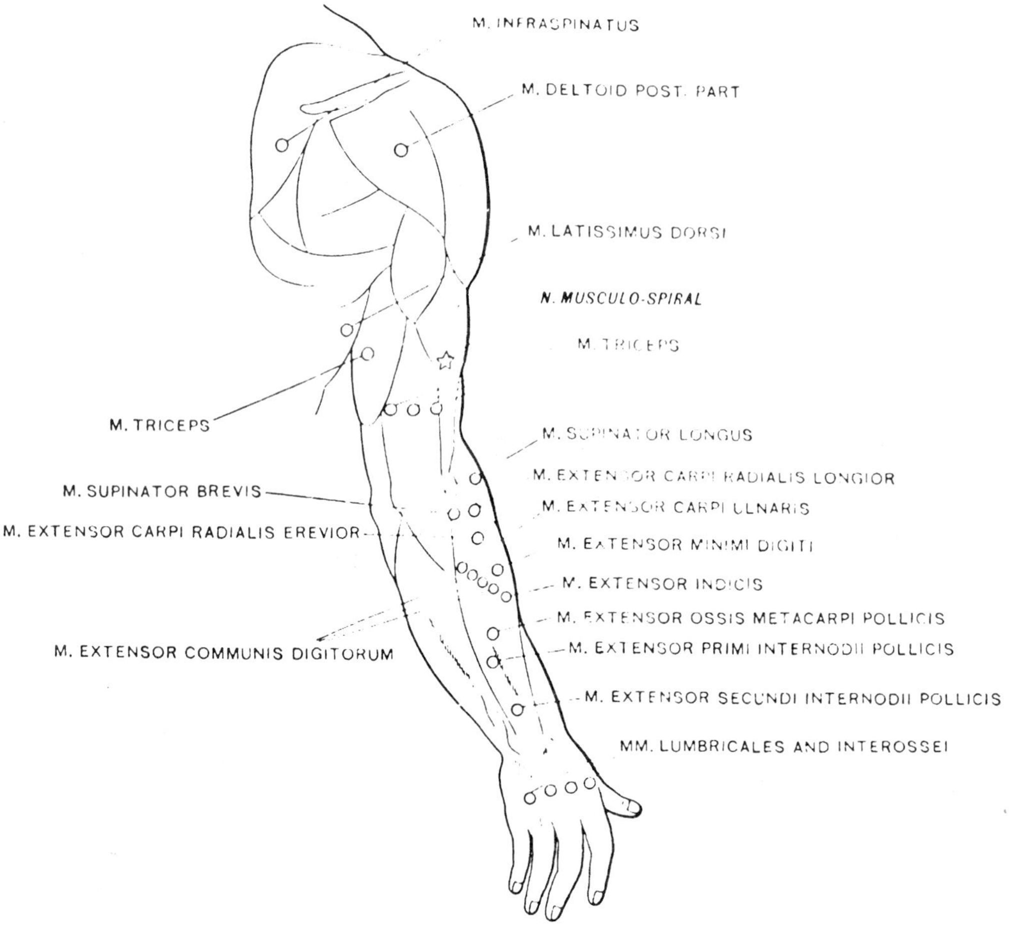

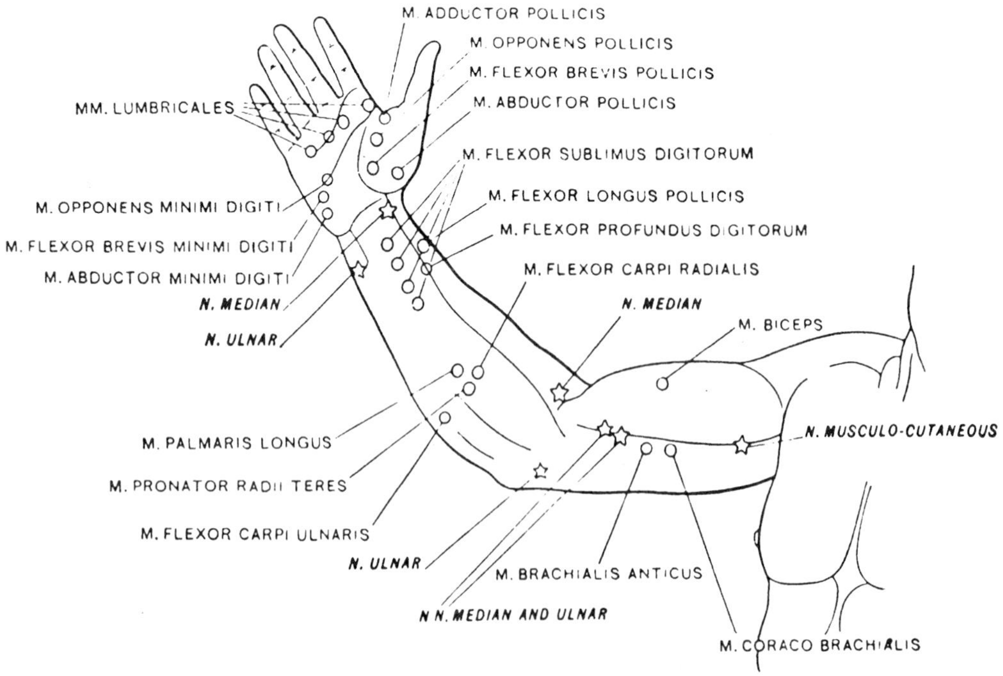

From Mettler Electronics® Corporation, Anaheim, California, with permission.

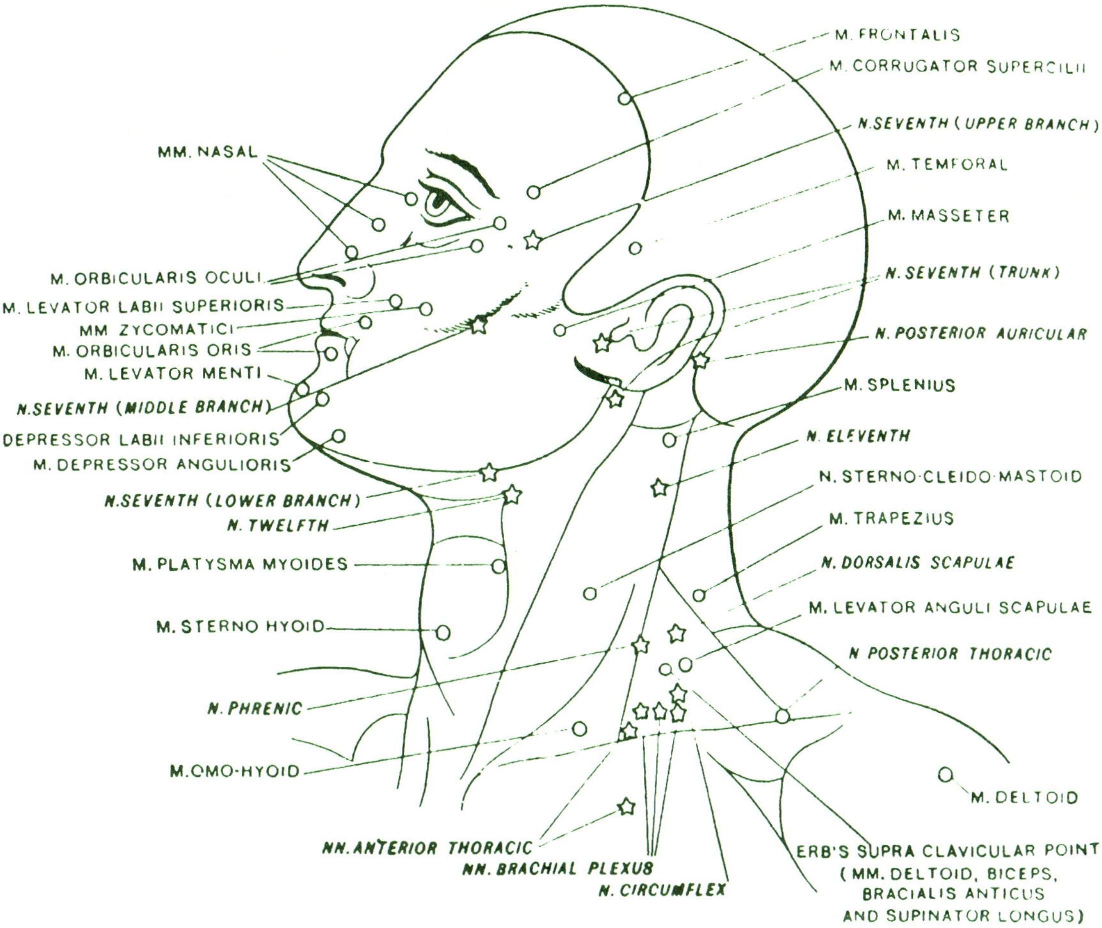

From Mettler Electronics® Corporation, Anaheim, California, with permission.

Acupuncture Points

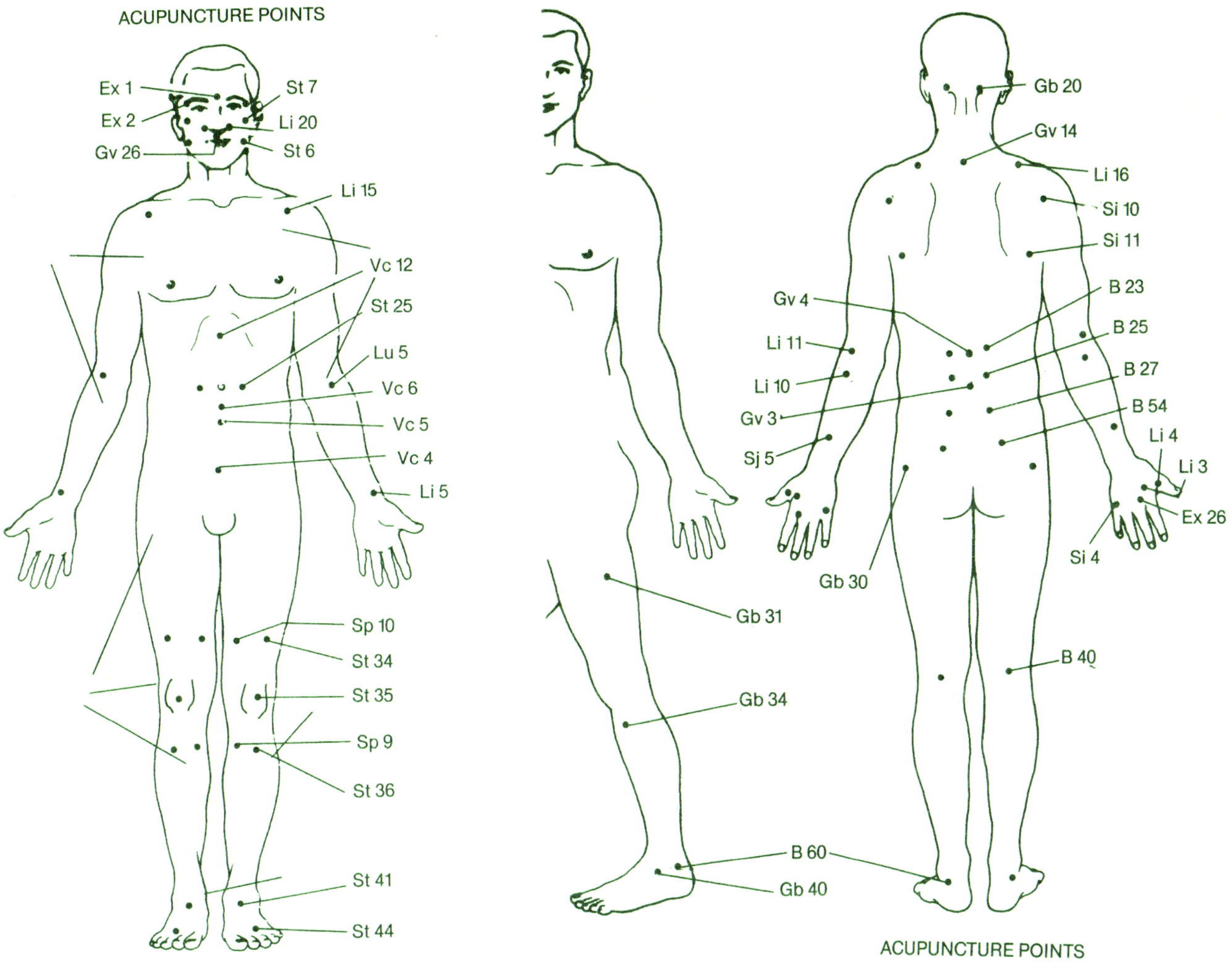

From Rothstein, JM, Roy, SH, and Wolf, SL: The Rehabilitation Specialist's Handbook. FA Davis, Philadelphia, 1991, pp 445, 446, with permission.

Appendix D

Interfacing Electrical Modalities with an Oscilloscope

A standard oscilloscope may be used to see the actual pulse form generated by various electrical modalities in various modes. As presented in Figure 17, two leads, one of the oscilloscope's active leads and its reference lead are spliced into one of the cables exiting the generator. The other active lead is connected to the cable of the modality. A 100- to 2000-ohm (Ω) resistor (available from an electronics supply store) is connected between the terminal ends of each of the modality's cables to roughly represent skin resistance. The oscilloscope's input parameters (e.g., amperage threshold and sweep rate) are then adjusted to the particular modality and its output parameters.

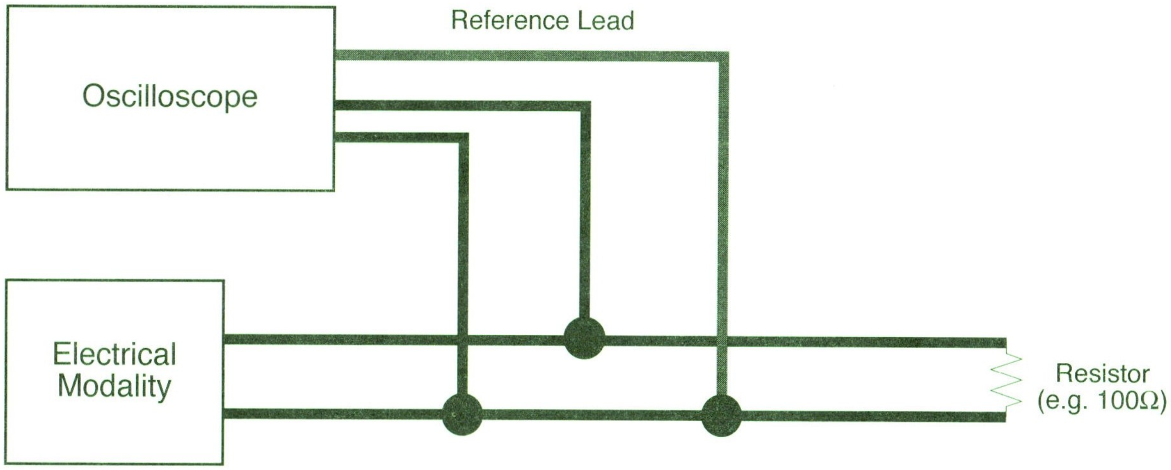

Figure 18. Interfacing an oscilloscope with an electrical stimulation unit.

After making the connections described above, turn on the oscilloscope and the modality. Fine tune the display so that the pulse's baseline is centered on the oscilloscope's grid and make other fine tuning adjustments as required. Modify the modality's output parameters and note the corresponding changes on the oscilloscope. When the output intensity is increased or decreased the height (amplitude) of the pulse will change correspondingly; increasing the pulse duration will cause the pulse to widen; increasing the number of pulses per second will increase the number of pulses displayed on the screen. Change modalities and notices the similarities and differences in the pulse shapes.

The benefits of this demonstration are largely dependent on the type of oscilloscope being used. Many advanced models have options to freeze the screen while others yet provide for printing the current image.

Assistance with and the materials needed for this project are often available through an engineering or physics department.

Answers to Activity Questions

Class Activity 1

1. The answer largely depends on the size of the cold modality and the temperature of the cold application. If the initial temperature of the treatment and the size of the delivery area are equal, those modalities having a wet medium have been shown to decrease skin surface temperature significantly.[9,10]

2. The redness (erythema) associated with cold application is thought to be attributed to a decreased dissociation of oxygen from hemoglobin at colder temperatures, making the superficial blood appear more red.[11] This effect could also be the result of local histamine release occurring from a local skin inflammatory response.

3. The answer is directly related to question 1 above. Those modalities producing the greatest skin temperature decrease will result in the greatest decrease in subcutaneous temperatures. In addition to being influenced by the availability of various forms of cold, the treatment of deep tissues requires a colder modality applied for a longer duration than the treatment of more superficial tissues. Keep in mind that adipose tissue serves as a barrier against cold penetration.

Class Activity 2

1. Although true anesthesia may never be obtained during ice immersion, analgesia does occur. This effect appears to be heightened because of the relative amount of pain experienced during the early minutes of immersion.

2. The digits appear to be the most sensitive to cold exposure, perhaps because of their small cross-section, relatively larger surface area, and the sensitivity of the lumina. Studies have indicated that the use of a neoprene covering over the toes greatly reduces the amount of perceived pain during this treatment[12] and that patients become habituated with repeated treatment.[13]

Class Activity 3

1. As we determined in Class Activity 1, wet ice tends to cool the skin more efficiently than "dry ice." Therefore, we would expect wet media to serve as a conductor in the transfer of cold, and dry media to serve as a skin insulator.

2. Insulating media are often incorrectly and overly used during the application of cold modalities. This well-intentioned safety measure often results in the overinsulation of the target tissues, negating any therapeutic effects.

Class Activity 4

1. As with cold, water serves as a conducting medium for the transfer of heat. Therefore, we would expect the greatest increases in skin temperature to occur with those modalities employing water. Like cold application, the result of thermotherapy greatly depends on the starting temperature of the modality, the size of the delivery area, and the duration of the treatment.

2. The skin begins to cool and return to its original temperature almost immediately after the removal of the heat source whereas cold has more latent effects. Heat application results in vasodilation, increasing the amount of cool blood delivered to the area, thus rapidly cooling the skin. Conversely, cold application and its associated vasoconstriction decrease the arrival of warm blood, yielding longer-lasting effects.

Class Activity 5

1. Although heat is commonly associated with increasing flexibility, the reduction of muscle spasm and reduced pain are effects of both cold and heat treatments. All of these factors may result in an increased range of motion following their application. In one study conducted in a manner similar to this activity, a significantly increased hip flexion range of motion was demonstrated after application of each modality.[14] The increase in range of motion was similar for both heat and cold.

2. For long-lasting increases in range of motion to occur, modality use must be augmented with or followed by flexibility exercises. Heat, because of its effect of increasing collagen extensibility and comfort, is often the modality of choice. A low-load prolonged stretch combined with heat application was found to produce a greater increase in shoulder external range of motion when compared with a low-load stretch alone.[15]

Class Activity 6

1. The hypertensive person should avoid extremes of temperature with full body immersion.

2. If the same temperatures were used, greater changes in blood pressure and temperature would be evident. In general, the greater the proportion of the body submerged during cold immersion, the greater the temperature of the water. The opposite is true with hot immersion; as more of the body is submerged, the temperature of the water decreases.

Class Activity 7

1. The longer the pulse duration, the less the interval between stimulation of sensory, motor, and pain fibers. In theory, all three types of fibers would be stimulated at the same time if the pulse duration were long enough and the intensity sufficient to cause a depolarization. This is what makes the use of a direct (galvanic) current uncomfortable.

2. A relatively short pulse duration would be better used when sensory stimulation alone is desired.

3. Much of the power of the stimulus is lost attempting to overcome the resistance offered by the skin-electrode interface. This reduction of power makes the actual energy delivered to the subcutaneous tissues significantly less than that indicated by the metered output. Proper measures used to decrease the resistance between the skin and the electrode, such as thoroughly covering the electrode with water or gel, cleaning the electrodes and skin, and ensuring the structural integrity of the electrode itself, help reduce the energy lost to resistance.

4. When this activity is concluded using the initial pulse duration, it would be expected that a greater output intensity is required to elicit sensory stimulation. The difference in intensity is explained by accommodation.

Class Activity 8

1. The same amount of current is flowing through the body whether the arm is submerged to level 5 or level 1. As the amount of skin surface area in contact with the water decreases, the current density increases geometrically. As the hand is withdrawn from the water, eventually the entire current would flow from the remaining finger tip, causing an inadvertent discovery of this concept.

2. To reduce sensation under the dispersive electrode: (a) increase the size of the dispersive electrode, (b) decrease the size of the active electrode(s), (c) ensure that the electrodes are thoroughly saturated with water or covered with conductive gel, (d) ensure that the dispersive electrode is in full contact with the body, (e) move the dispersive electrode to another body part to reduce the effects of body hair resisting current flow.

Class Activity 9

1. As you can see from the chart, motor points tend to be found over the belly of the muscle.[16] A chart provides a motor point's approximate placement, but its exact location is unique to each individual and can vary for the same person over time.

2. As previously described, Pfleuger's law describes that muscle contraction occurs more comfortably and at a lower intensity under the cathode (negative pole) than under the anode. Many neuromuscular electrical stimulation units use a biphasic pulse, illustrating the minimal influence of this property without a long or continuous pulse duration.

3. Yes, although a higher current intensity will be required for depolarization to occur. Incidentally, the muscle fiber itself (as opposed to the motor nerve) can be electrically stimulated to fire given that a long (> 1 msec) pulse duration or galvanic current is used. Stimulators that can achieve these properties are used to elicit contractions from denervated muscle.

Class Activity 10

1. If you used the same partner, the motor point should have been in the same location for this exercise; however, because you might not have been able to tolerate an intensity sufficient for stimulation of motor points, muscle activity may have not been evident.

2. As mentioned in the previous response, the maximal output intensity is most probably limited by what your finger can tolerate as an electrode. An increased current density is experienced at the electrode with the smaller surface area — your finger in this case.

Class Activity 11

1. In this activity, the current is more concentrated at the target muscle using the bipolar electrode arrangement, resulting in a stronger contraction. Because the dispersive electrode is away from the target area with a monopolar arrangement, the current's path includes many parallel circuits, diminishing its strength at the desired muscle.

2. A tonic contraction is achieved with neuromuscular electrical stimulation at a frequency of between 35 and 50 pps. Frequencies beyond this range result in greater muscle tension developed at the expense of increased muscular fatigue.[17]

3. As you have seen, both a high-volt electrical stimulator and a neuromuscular electrical stimulator (NMES) can be used to elicit muscle contractions, although NMES does so more efficiently. The NMES stimulator is thought to be better for eliciting muscle contractions because its biphasic wave form is better tolerated, allowing for greater current to be applied with less discomfort.

4. Electrically induced muscle contractions fatigue more quickly than strictly voluntary contractions, possibly because of changes in motor fiber recruitment patterns. Because of this, a duty cycle is routinely incorporated into neuromuscular re-education, with the most studied "OFF" time being 50 seconds.[18] The longer the OFF time, the more time for muscular recovery is allowed.

Class Activity 12

1. Because ice is known to slow nerve conduction velocity and subsequently reduce pain, an increased tolerance of electrical current would be expected. This presumes that electrically induced pain is experienced at a superficial level.

2. Ice massage has been demonstrated to increase blood flow. This effect may have decreased the level of resistance within the muscle, thus improving the current's efficiency.

Class Activity 13

No activity questions.

Class Activity 14

1. Gel tends to be the best medium for transmitting ultrasound because of its high concentration of salt-free water.

2. Thick cream is not a good conductor of ultrasonic energy, especially when mixed with corticosteroid.[8]

3. Some mixtures of phonophoresis cream, especially low doses of hydrocortisone, allow a small percentage of ultrasonic energy to pass through the sound head. This fact, coupled with a limited ability of these creams to be absorbed through the skin, may have permitted a sufficient quantity of the medication to be introduced into the body.

Class Activity 15

1. Some individuals respond best to auditory feedback when attempting to increase muscular strength, presumably because it allows them to focus visually on the contracting muscle. However, the total torque production should have been greatest in either group using feedback.

2. Biofeedback implies that some process occurring in the body is being measured and related back to the individual in a usable manner. Yelling encouragement or touching the muscle to facilitate contractions are examples of external feedback. Both techniques, used either individually or jointly, will assist in the education of muscle.

Class Activity 16

1. This effect supports the concept of bilateral transfer, where the contraction of a muscle or muscle group results in the "spilling" of impulses to the contralateral side. A technique used in re-educating muscle is to have the individual attempt to contract muscles bilaterally.

2. To assist with muscular relaxation, reverse the process just followed. Set the threshold at the level where muscle activity is detected and gradually lower it so that the unit becomes more sensitive to changes in electrical activity. The instructions to the user are to turn the sound off by relaxing the particular muscle.

   Whenever possible, biofeedback training should be conducted in a quiet room, especially during relaxation training. Additionally, when a biofeedback unit is being used for muscular relaxation, a soothing, low-pitched auditory feedback sound is preferred.

Class Activity 17

1-2. The efficiency of traction is based on: (a) the force of gravity, (b) friction, and (c) the angle of pull.

Appendix F

Answers to Class Exercises

Class Exercise 1

1. A - In a series circuit, the total resistance is equal to the sum of the resistors:

   $R_t = r_1 + r_2 + r_3$

   R_t = 20 ohms + 30 ohms + 40 ohms

   R_t = 90 ohms

   B - In a parallel circuit, the total resistance is equal to the reciprocal of the sum of the resistors:

   $1/R_t = 1/r_1 + 1/r_2 + 1/r_3$

   $1/R_t$ = 1/20 ohms + 1/30 ohms + 1/40 ohms

   $1/R_t = 0.050 + 0.033 + 0.025$

   $1/R_t = 0.108$

   $R_t = 1/0.108$

   R_t = 9.26 ohms

2. Amperage is calculated by the equation $I = V/R_t$:

   A - The amperage in the series circuit is calculated by:

   $I = V/R_t$

   I = 120 volts/90 ohms (obtained from question 1-A)

   I = 1.3 amperes

   B - The amperage in the parallel circuit is calculated by:

   $I = V/R_t$

   I = 120 Volts / 9.26 Ohms (obtained from question 1-B)

   I = 13 amperes (12.959 rounded up)

3. A -

   $I = V/R_t$

   I = 200 volts / 90 ohms

   I = 2.22 amperes

B -

$I = V/R_t$

I = 200 volts / 9.26 ohms

I = 21.6 amperes

4. Wattage is calculated by multiplying the voltage by the amperage (W = VI):

A -

W = VI

W = 120 volts x 1.3 amperes

W = 156 watts

B -

W = VI

W = 120 volts x 13 amperes

W = 1,560 watts

5. In a series circuit, the voltage across each resistor is calculated by:

Resistor 1	Resistor 2	Resistor 3
$V_1 = Ir_1$	$V_2 = Ir_2$	$V_3 = Ir_3$
V_1 = 10 amperes x 20 ohms	V_2 = 10 amperes x 30 ohms	V_3 = 10 amperes x 40 ohms
V_1 = 200 Volts	V_2 = 300 Volts	V_3 = 400 Volts

6. In a parallel circuit, amperage across each path is calculated by:

Resistor 1	Resistor 2	Resistor 3
$I_1 = V/R_1$	$I_2 = V/R_2$	$I_3 = V/R_3$
I_1 = 100 volts/20 ohms	I_2 = 100 volts/30 ohms	I_3 = 100 Volts/40 Ohms
I_1 = 5 amperes	I_2 = 3.3 amperes	I_3 = 2.5 amperes

7. The total resistance is calculated by:

$1/R_t = 1/r_1 + 1/r_2 + 1/r_3 + 1/r_4 + 1/r_5$

$1/R_t$ = 1/20 ohms + 1/30 ohms + 1/40 ohms + 1/30 ohms + 1/30 ohms

$1/R_t = 0.050 + 0.033 + 0.025 + 0.033 + 0.033$

$1/R_t = 0.174$

$R_t = 1/0.174$

R_t = 5.75 ohms

8. Amperage is calculated by the equation:

$I = V/R_t$

I = 120 / 5.75 ohms

I = 20.9 amperes

9. As resistors are added to a parallel circuit the total resistance decreases (compare your answers from questions 1-B and 7). As you will recall, amperage is related to the reciprocal of the resistance provided. Therefore as resistance is added, current flow increases.

Class Exercise 2

1. A

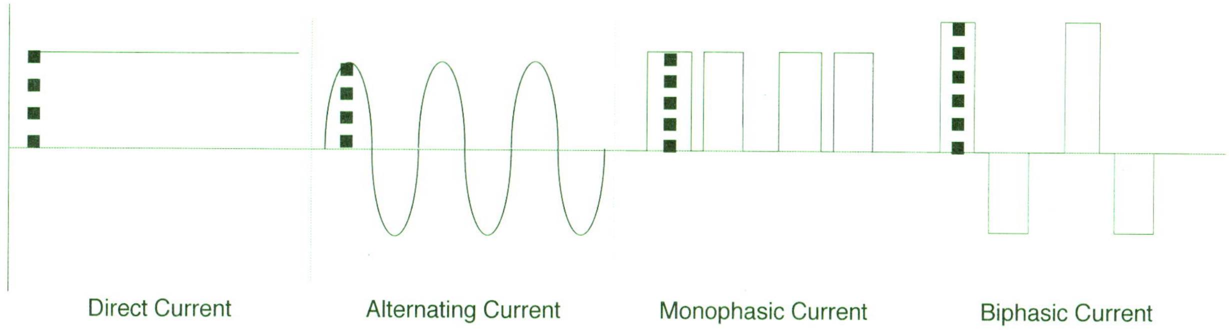

B

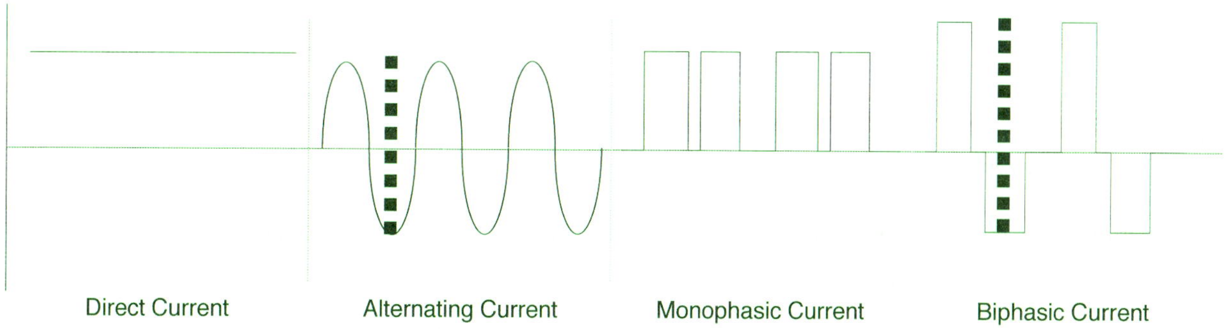

C

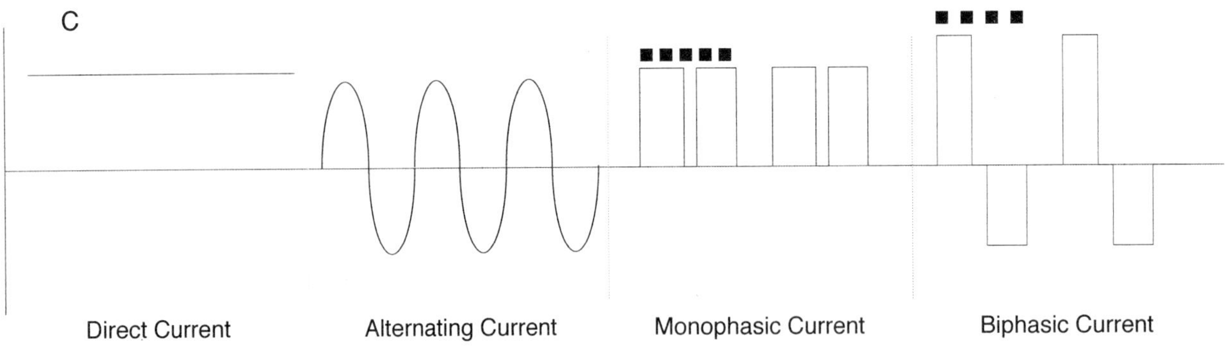

There is no pulse duration for direct currents and alternating currents because they are not pulsed.

D

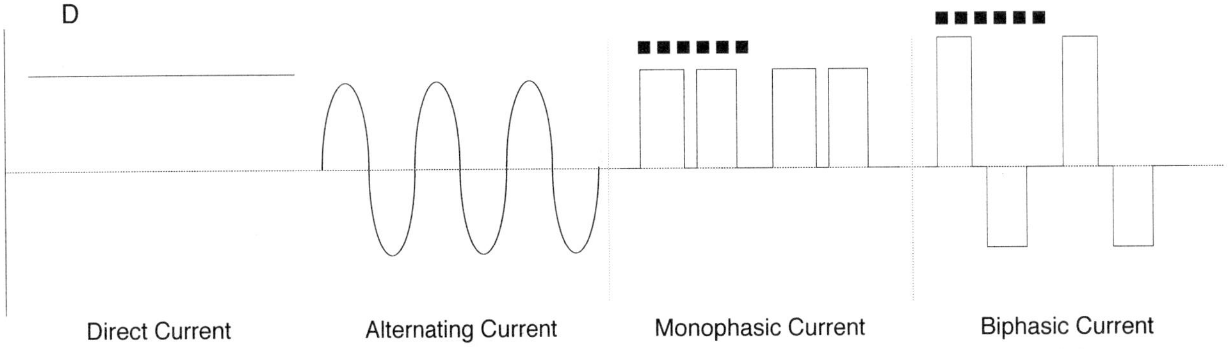

There is no pulse period for direct currents and alternating currents because they are not pulsed.

E

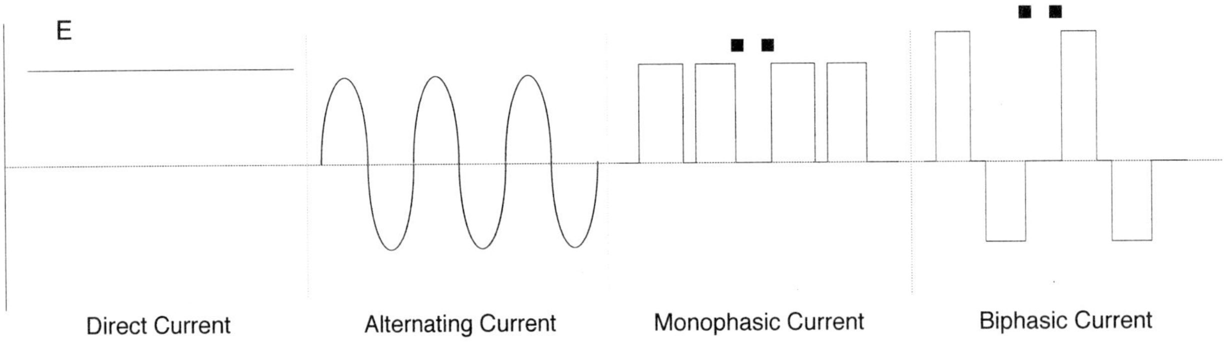

There is no interpulse interval for the direct current and alternating current because they are not pulsed.

F

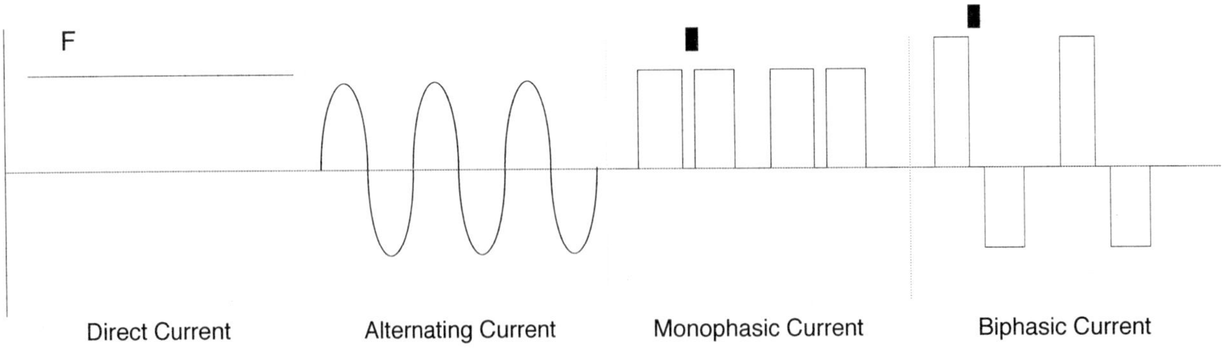

There is no intrapulse interval for direct currents and alternating currents because they are not pulsed.

2. The answer is found by first finding how long the current flows during 1 second (pulse duration x pulses per second) and then multiplying that figure by 60 seconds:

Current flow/second = pulse duration x pulses per second

Current flow/second = 140 μsec x 125 pps

Current flow/second = 0.0001 second x 125 pps

Current flow/second = 0.0175 second

Current flow/minute = (current flow/second x 60 seconds)

Current flow/minute = 0.0175 second x 60 Sec

Current flow/minute = 1.05 seconds

3. The pulse charge, measured in coulombs, may be increased or decreased by increasing or decreasing the amplitude, pulse duration, or both (see Appendix D, Interfacing Electrical Modalities with an Oscilloscope).

Class Exercise 3

1. The maximal output within an ultrasound beam is calculated by multiplying the beam nonuniformity ratio (BNR) by the metered output:

Maximal output = BNR x Metered Output

Maximal output = 4:1 x 4 watts

Maximal output = 16 watts

2. The spatial average intensity (SAI) is calculated by dividing the output (in watts) by the effective radiating area (ERA) of the sound head:

SAI = W/ERA

10 cm^2/5 Watts	=	2 W/cm^2
8 cm^2/5 Watts	=	1.6 W/cm^2
5 cm^2/5 Watts	=	1 W/cm^2
3 cm^2/5 Watts	=	0.6 W/cm^2
1 cm^2/5 Watts	=	0.2 W/cm^2

3. The percent duty cycle is calculated by the equation provided below. The temporal average intensity is calculated by multiplying the metered output by the percent duty cycle:

   Duty cycle = pulse duration/(pulse duration + pulse interval) x 100

% Duty Cycle	Temporal Average Intensity
10/(10 + 10) x 100 = 50%	4 W/cm^2 x 0.5 = 2 W/cm^2
20/(20 + 40) x 100 = 33%	4 W/cm^2 x 0.33 = 1.32 W/cm^2
10/(10 + 50) x 100 = 17%	4 W/cm^2 x 0.17 = 0.68 W/cm^2
25/(25 + 50) x 100 = 33%	4 W/cm^2 x 0.33 = 1.32 W/cm^2

Appendix G

Problems Derived from Case Studies

Case Study 1

Problems:

1. Decreased ROM
2. Pain
3. Potential to form myositis ossificans
4. Localized swelling

Case Study 2

Problems:

1. Pain
2. Decreased function/strength
3. Swelling
4. Active inflammatory process

Case Study 3

Problems:

1. Decreased ROM due to capsular tightness
2. Biomechanical changes in scapulohumeral function
3. Decreased function of left shoulder
4. Minimal complaints of pain

Case Study 4

Problems:

1. Inability to perform quadriceps contraction
2. Decreased ROM
3. Disuse atrophy
4. Extension lag
5. Minimal complaints of pain

Case Study 5

Problems:

1. Pain, especially in the evening
2. Glenohumeral instability
3. Overuse injury - activity can be modified, but training cannot be interrupted

Case Study 6

Problems:

1. Effusion
2. Decreased patellar mobility
3. Decreased ROM
4. Minimal complaints of pain

Case Study 7

Problems:

1. Decreased ROM
2. Gait alteration
3. Pitting edema
4. Mild pain

Case Study 8

Problems:

1. Decreased ROM
2. Tight hamstrings

Additional Workbook Grids

The following grids are copies of those used in the exercises. The student can tear them out and record findings while still looking at the procedures, submit the exercises to the instructor, or retain an extra copy in the event of a mistake.

Skin Temperature Decrease Worksheet

Name: ____________________ Date: ____________

Partner(s): ______________________________

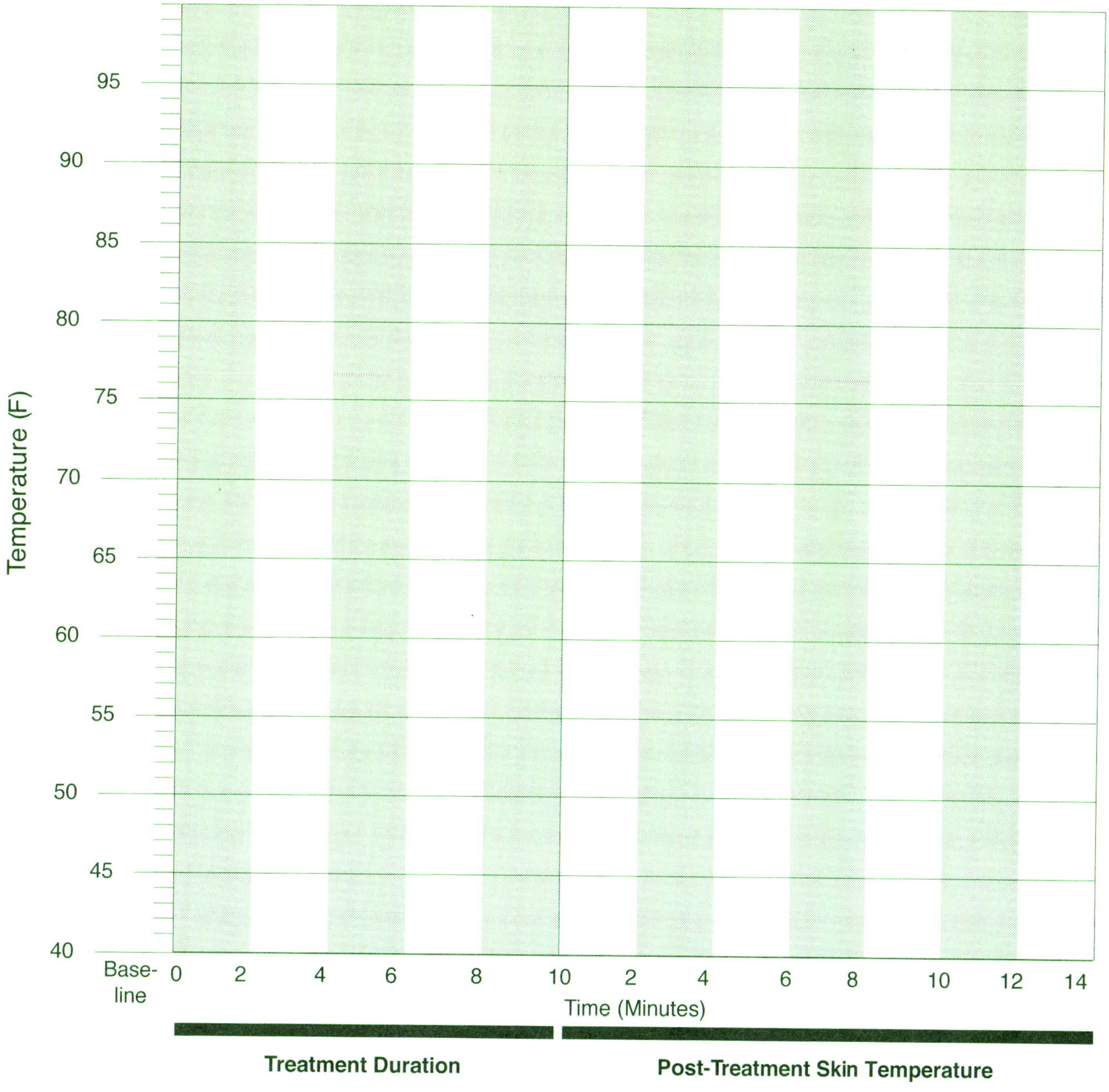

Labeling Key			
○	Crushed Ice Bag	△	Instant Cold Pack
●	Ice Immersion	▲	Vapocoolant Spray
□	Ice Massage	X	Other:
■	Reusable Cold Pack		Other:

Pain Perception During Ice Immersion Worksheet

Name: ______________________ Date: ____________

Partner(s): ____

1 Minute Post-Immersion

No Pain — Worst Pain Imaginable

0 1 2 3 4 5 6 7 8 9 10

3 Minutes Post-Immersion

No Pain — Worst Pain Imaginable

0 1 2 3 4 5 6 7 8 9 10

5 Minutes Post-Immersion

No Pain — Worst Pain Imaginable

0 1 2 3 4 5 6 7 8 9 10

7 Minutes Post-Immersion

No Pain — Worst Pain Imaginable

0 1 2 3 4 5 6 7 8 9 10

9 Minutes Post-Immersion

No Pain — Worst Pain Imaginable

0 1 2 3 4 5 6 7 8 9 10

11 Minutes Post-Immersion

No Pain — Worst Pain Imaginable

0 1 2 3 4 5 6 7 8 9 10

Plot of Pain Perception Over Time

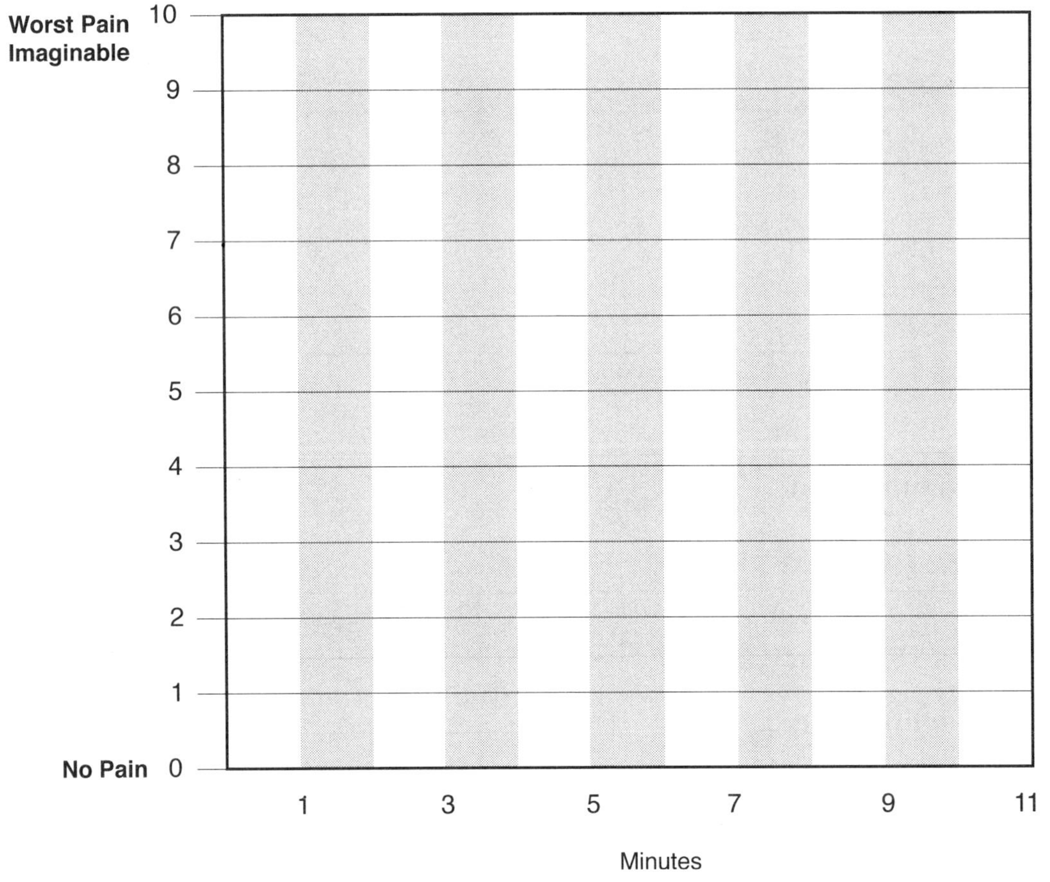

Labeling Key	
■	No Toe Cap
●	With Toe Cap

Effects of Insulating Media on Skin Temperature Decrease Worksheet

Name: ______________________ Date: ______________

Partner(s): ____

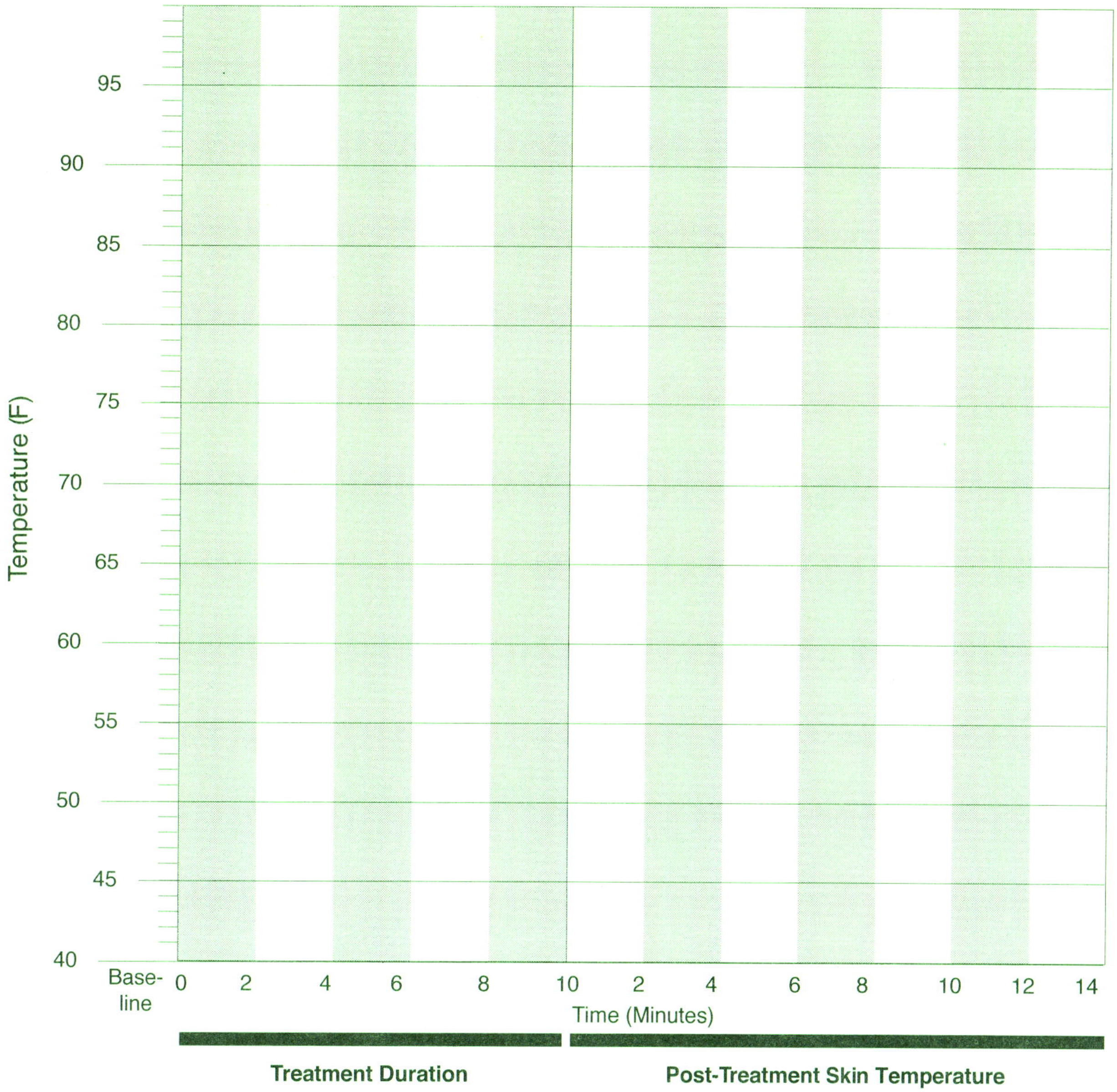

Labeling Key			
○	Wet Elastic Wrap	■	No Insulation (From Activity 1)
●	Dry Terry Cloth	△	Other
□	Damp Terry Cloth	▲	Other

Skin Temperature Increase Worksheet

Name: ______________________ Date: __________

Partner(s): ______________________________________

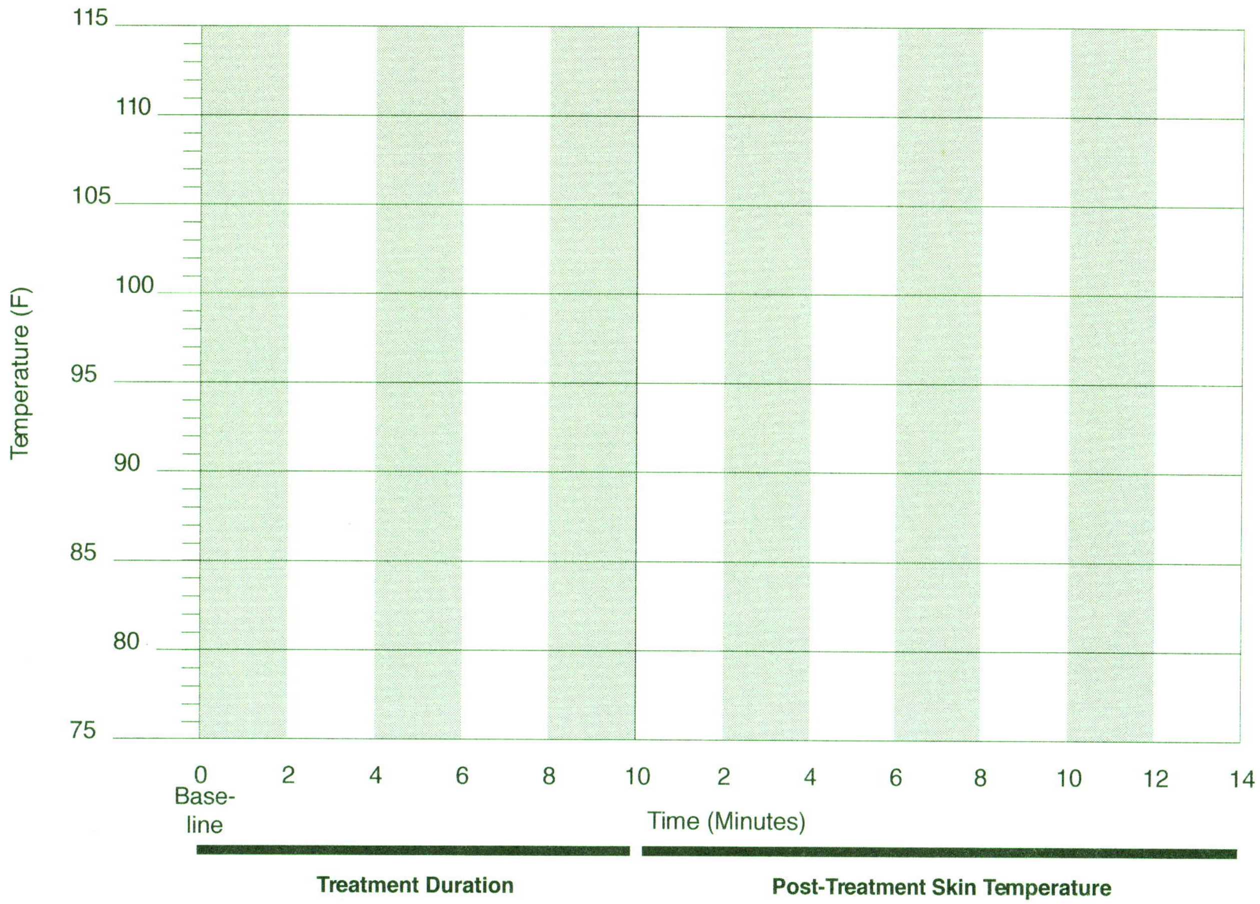

Labeling Key			
○	Moist Heat Pack	■	Warm Water Immersion
●	Dry Heat	△	Other
□	Paraffin	▲	Other

Effect of Heat and Cold on Tissue Elasticity Worksheet

Name: ______________________ Date: ______________

Partner(s): ______________________________________

Hamstring ROM Measurement Used: ☐ Sit-and-Reach ☐ Goniometer
☐ Stand-and-Reach ☐ Other: ____________

Subject	Modality Used	Pre-Test	Post-Test
	☐ Heat ☐ Cold		
	☐ Heat ☐ Cold		
	☐ Heat ☐ Cold		
	☐ Heat ☐ Cold		
	☐ Heat ☐ Cold		

Composite Scores:

Cold Application			
Subject	Pre	Post	Diff
Net Change			

Heat Application			
Subject	Pre	Post	Diff
Net Change			

Effect of Heat and Cold on Pulse and Blood Pressure Worksheet

Name: ____________________ Date: ____________

Partner(s): ______________________________

Type of Modality Used: ☐ Heat ☐ Cold

Test Measurements:

		During Application					Post-Application				
	Baseline	2	4	6	8	10	2	4	6	8	10
Pulse											
Blood Pressure											

Plot of Changes in Blood Pressure and Pulse Rate

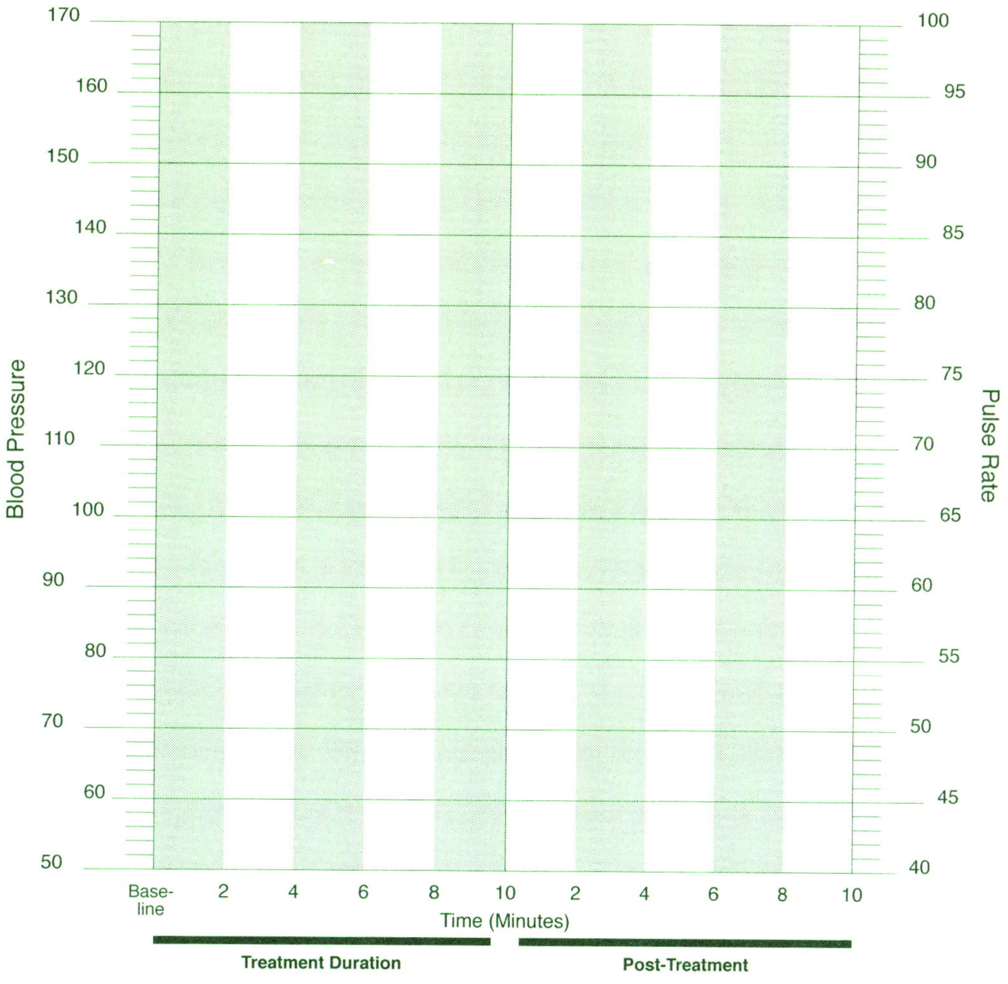

Labeling Key			
Blood Pressure (left axis)			Pulse Rate (right axis)
●	Systolic Pressure	■	Pulse Rate
○	Diastolic Pressure		

Type of Modality Used: ☐ Heat ☐ Cold

Test Measurements:

	Baseline	During Application 2	4	6	8	10	Post-Application 2	4	6	8	10
Pulse											
Blood Pressure											

Plot of Changes in Blood Pressure and Pulse Rate

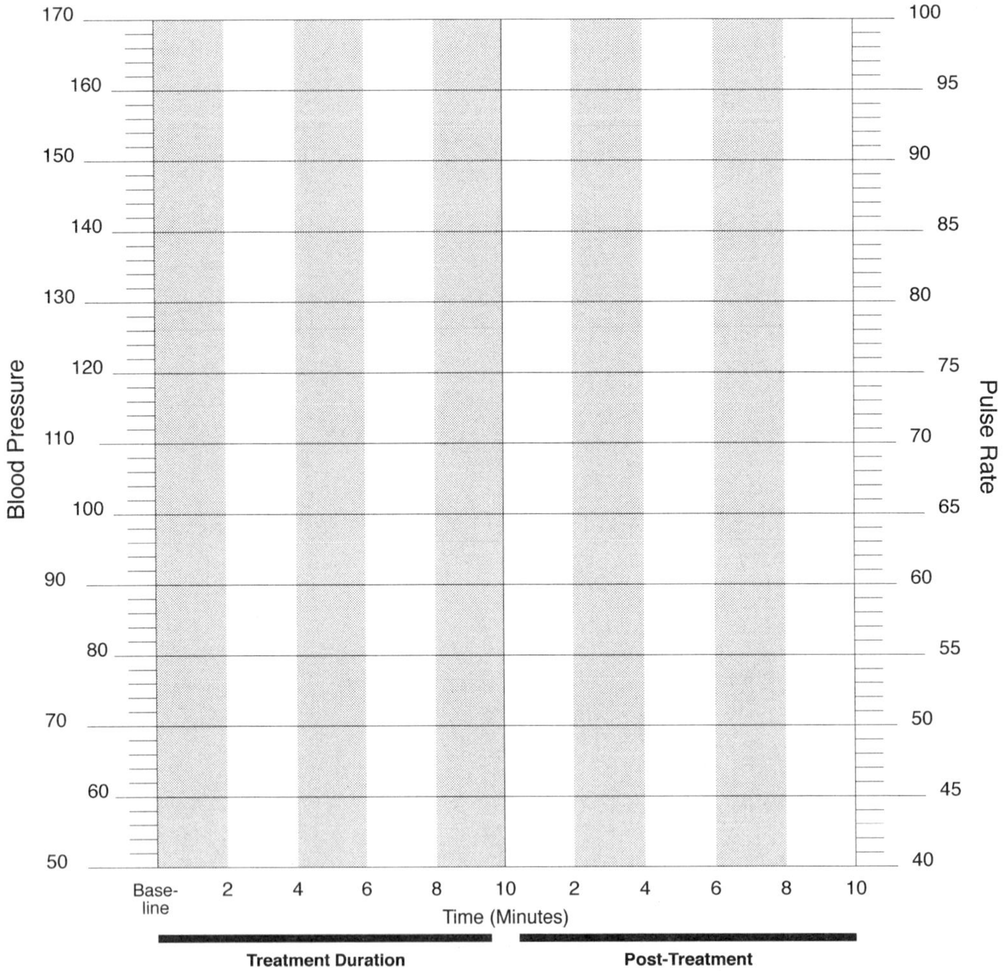

Labeling Key			
	Blood Pressure (left axis)		Pulse Rate (right axis)
●	Systolic Pressure	■	Pulse Rate
○	Diastolic Pressure		

Selective Stimulation of Nerves Worksheet

Name: ____________________ Date: __________

Partner(s): ____________________

Type of Stimulation Unit Used: ____________________

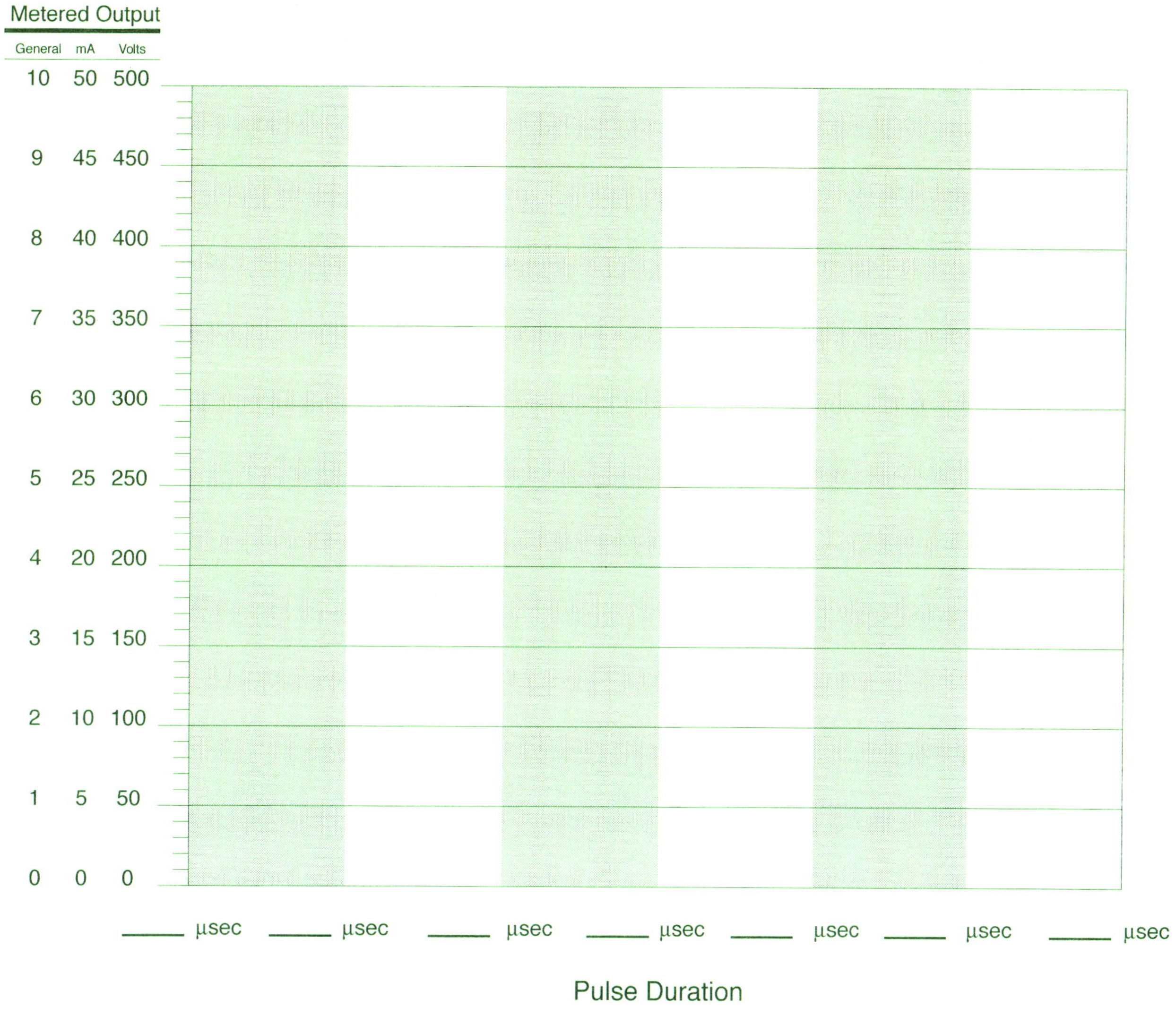

Labeling Key	
●	Sensory Nerves
○	Motor Nerves
□	Pain Nerves

Current Density Worksheet

Name: ______________________ Date: ____________

Partner(s): ______________________________________

Type of Stimulation Unit Used: ______________________________

Stimulus Perception at the Level "5" Mark

No Sensation — **Intolerable Sensation**

0 1 2 3 4 5 6 7 8 9 10

Stimulus Perception at the Level "4" Mark

No Sensation — **Intolerable Sensation**

0 1 2 3 4 5 6 7 8 9 10

Stimulus Perception at the Level "3" Mark

No Sensation — **Intolerable Sensation**

0 1 2 3 4 5 6 7 8 9 10

Stimulus Perception at the Level "2" Mark

No Sensation — **Intolerable Sensation**

0 1 2 3 4 5 6 7 8 9 10

Stimulus Perception at the Level "1" Mark

No Sensation — **Intolerable Sensation**

0 1 2 3 4 5 6 7 8 9 10

Identification of Motor Points Worksheet

Name: ______________________ Date: ____________

Partner(s): ______________________________________

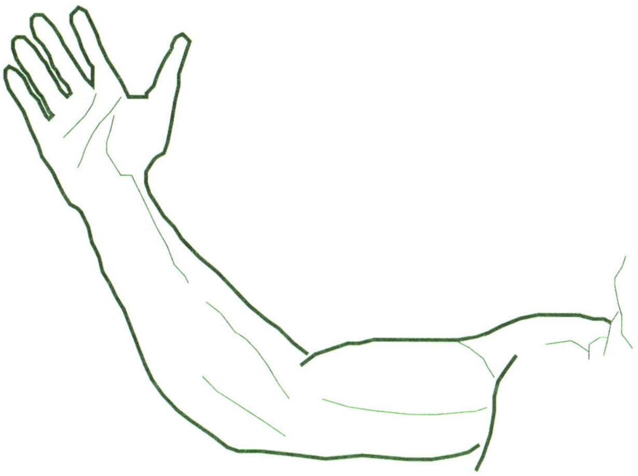

Arm - Anterior View

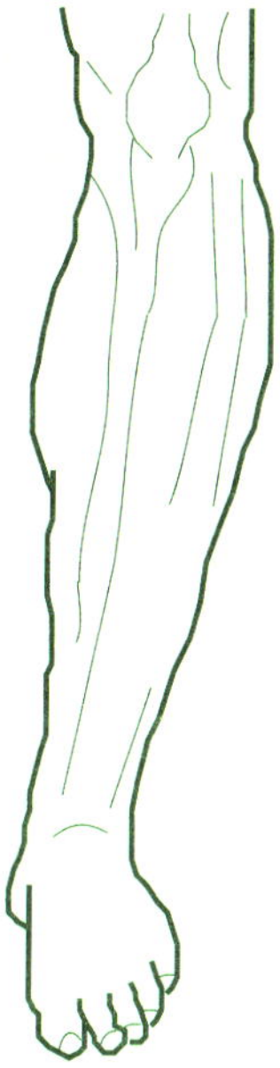

Leg - Anterior View

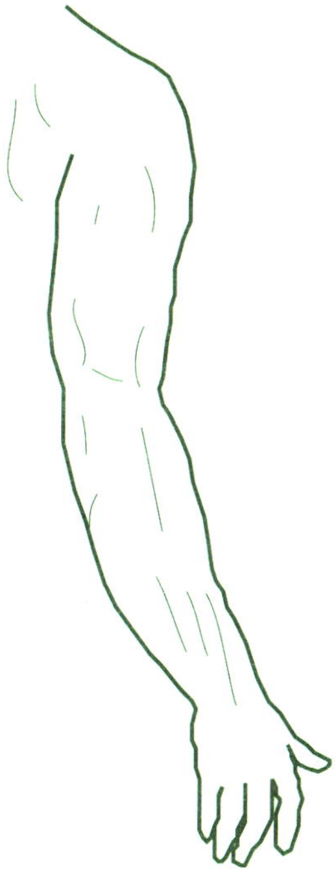

Arm - Posterior View

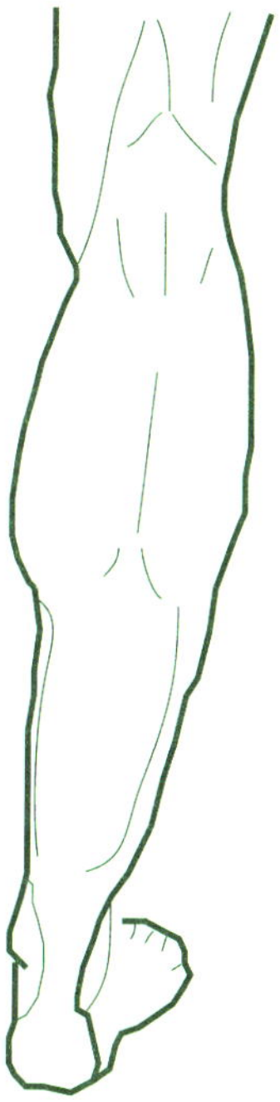

Leg - Posterior View

(Labeling key on reverse)

Labeling Key

Upper Extremity

1 Abductor pollicis
2 Extensor digiti minimi
3 Extensor indicis
4 Flexor carpi radialis
5 Flexor carpi ulnaris

6 Other: ______

7 Other: ______

8 Other: ______

9 Other: ______

10 Other: ______

Lower Extremity

A Abductor digiti minimi
B Extensor hallucis longus
C Peroneus longus
D Extensor digitorum brevis
E Tibialis anterior

F Other: ______

G Other: ______

H Other: ______

I Other: ______

J Other: ______

Manual Determination of Optimal Stimulation Sites Worksheet

Name: ______________________ Date: ______________

Partner(s): ______________________________________

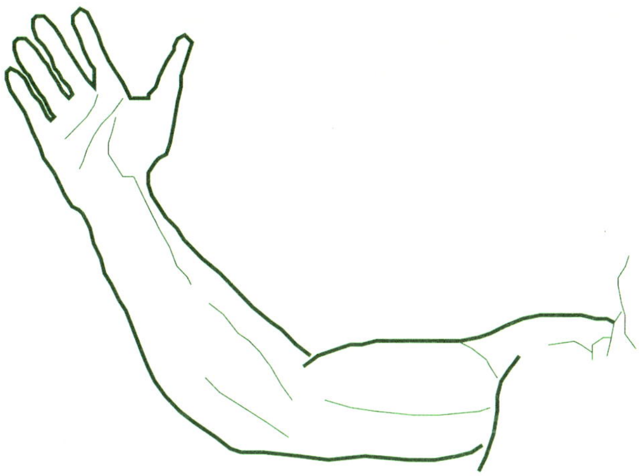

Arm - Anterior View

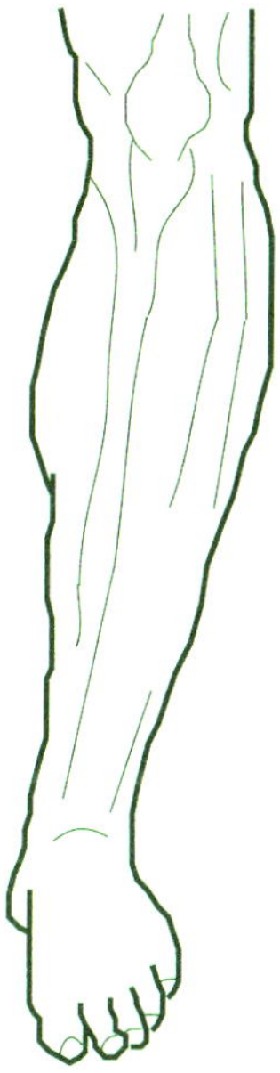

Leg - Anterior View

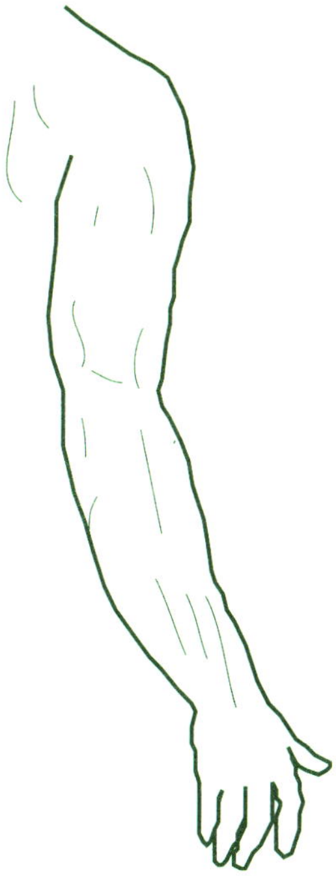

Arm - Posterior View

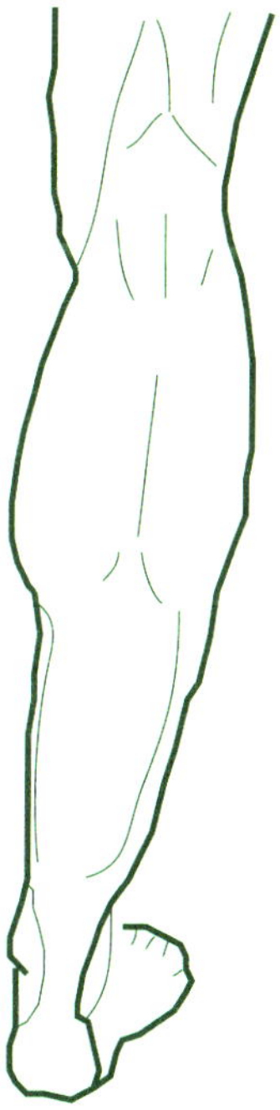

Leg - Posterior View

Labeling Key	
○ No Associated Muscle Contraction	● Muscle Contraction Associated

Strength of Electrically Elicited Muscle Contractions Worksheet

Name: ______________________ Date: ______________

Partner(s): ______________________________________

Baseline Torque Production:

Maximal Voluntary Isometric Contraction	
Joint Angle	Peak Torque

Involuntary Torque Production:

Electrical Stimulator	Electrode Configuration	Pulse Duration	Pulses per Second	Duty Cycle	Max. Output Intensity	Joint Angle	Peak Torque	% MVIC

Effect of Cold Application in Reducing the Perception of Electrically Induced Pain Worksheet

Name: ______________________ Date: ____________

Partner(s): ____

Subject	Maximum Output Intensity No Cold Application	With Cold Application	Difference

Coupling Ability of Various Ultrasound Media Worksheet

Name: ______________________ Date: ______________

Partner(s): ____

ERA of sound head:

Coupling Medium	Watts Needed to Cause "Bubbles"

ERA of sound head:

Coupling Medium	Watts Needed to Cause "Bubbles"

Strength of Biofeedback-Augmented Muscle Contractions Worksheet

Name: ____________________ Date: ____________

Partner(s): ______________________________________

Subject	Maximum Voluntary Contraction Force Produced			
	No Feedback (%)	Visual Feedback (%)	Audio Feedback (%)	Both (%)

Supine vs. Sitting Cervical Traction Worksheet

Name: ____________________ Date: ____________

Partner(s): ____

	Force Required			% of Dummy Weight		
Weight	Vertical	Horizontal		Vertical	Horizontal	% Difference
20 lbs.						

Modality Contraindications

Many of the activities described in this workbook require the application of a modality to a subject. Do not assume that your subject is free of contraindications to the use of these forms of energy. Listed below are the commonly accepted contraindications to the modalities included in this workbook.

Cold Modalities

- cardiac or respiratory involvement
- uncovered open wounds
- circulatory insufficiency
- cold allergy
- anesthetic skin
- Raynaud's phenomenon
- presence of regenerating peripheral nerves

Heat Modalities

- acute injuries
- impaired circulation
- poor thermal regulation
- anesthetic areas
- already existing fever
- malignancies
- cardiac insufficiency
- extremely old adults and children younger than 4 years old.

Electrical Stimulation

General

- cardiac disability
- exposed metal implants such as those used for external fixation
- severe obesity
- areas of particular sensitivity
  - carotid sinus
  - esophagus (laryngeal or pharyngeal muscles)
  - pharynx
  - mucosal membranes
- during pregnancy
- skin irritation due to electrode placement

Motor Level Stimulation

- unwanted muscle contraction or active movement
- hemorrhage or active inflammation
- malignancies

Direct Current (Ion Transfer)

- anesthetic skin
- recent scars
- metal implants
- acute injury
- cardiac pacemakers

Ultrasound

- acute conditions (continuous output)
- ischemic areas
- tendency to hemorrhage
- around the eyes, heart, skull, or genitals
- pregnancy when used over the pelvis or lumbar areas
- cancer
- over the spinal cord (post-laminectomy) or large nerve plexus (i.e., carotid sinus) in high doses
- anesthetic areas
- over a fracture site before healing is complete
- stress fracture sites
- active infection
- over the pelvic or lumbar areas in menstruating females
- areas of impaired circulation

Biofeedback

- contraindications are the same as for active exercise

References

1. Weinberger, A and Lev, A: Temperature elevation of connective tissue by physical modalities. Critical Reviews in Physical Rehabilitation Medicine 3:121, 1991.

2. Watkins, MP: Clinical evaluation of thermal agents. In Michlovitz, SL (ed): Thermal Agents in Rehabilitation, ed 2. FA Davis, Philadelphia, 1990, pp 221-244.

3. Arnheim, DD and Prentice, WE: Principles of Athletic Training, ed 8. Mosby, St. Louis, 1993, pp 308-346.

4. Ingersoll, CD and Mangus, BC: Sensations of cold reexamined: A study using the McGill Pain Questionnaire. Journal of Athletic Training 26:240,1991.

5. Nelson, RM and Currier, DP: Electrical stimulation of healthy muscle and tissue repair. In Nelson, RM and Currier, DP (eds): Clinical Electrotherapy, ed 2. Appleton & Lange, Norwalk, CT, 1991, pp 106-107.

6. Miller, CR and Webers, RL: The effects of ice massage on an individual's pain tolerance level to electrical stimulation. JOSPT 12:105, 1990.

7. Durst, JW, et al.: Effects of ice and recovery time on maximal involuntary isometric torque production using electrical stimulation. JOSPT 13:240, 1991.

8. Cameron, MH and Monroe, LG: Relative transmission of ultrasound by media customarily used for phonophoresis. Phys Ther 72:142, 1992.

9. Belitsky, RB, Odam, SJ, and Hubley-Kozey, C: Evaluation of the effectiveness of wet ice, dry ice, and cryogen packs in reducing skin temperature. Phys Ther 67:1080, 1987.

10. Bocobo, C, et al.: The effect of ice on intra-articular temperature in the knee of the dog. Am J Phys Med Rehabil 70:181, 1991.

11. Michlovitz, SL: Cryotherapy: The use of cold as a therapeutic agent. In Michlovitz, SL (ed): Thermal Agents in Rehabilitation, ed 2. FA Davis, Philadelphia, 1990, pp 63-84.

12. Nimchick, PSR and Knight, KL: Effects of wearing a toe cap or sock on temperature and perceived pain during ice immersion. Journal of Athletic Training 18:144, 1983.

13. Ingersoll, CD and Mangus, BC: Habituation to the perception of the qualities of cold-induced pain. Journal of Athletic Training 27:218, 1992.

14. Minton, J: A comparison of thermotherapy and cryotherapy in enhancing supine, extended-leg hip flexion. Journal of Athletic Training 28:172, 1993.

15. Lentell, G, et al.: The use of thermal agents to influence the effectiveness of a low-load prolonged stretch. JOSPT 16:200, 1992.

16. DeLitto, A and Robinson, AJ: Electrical stimulation of muscle: Techniques and applications. In Snyder-Mackler, L and Robinson, AJ (eds): Clinical Electrophysiology: Electrotherapy and Electrophysiologic Testing. Williams & Wilkins, Baltimore, 1989, p 102.

17. Hooker, DN: Electrical stimulating currents. In Prentice, W (ed): Therapeutic Modalities in Sports Medicine. Times Mirror/Mosby, St. Louis, 1990, p 61.

18. DeLitto, A and Robinson, AJ: Electrical stimulation of muscle: Techniques and applications. In Snyder-Mackler, L and Robinson, AJ (eds): Clinical Electrophysiology: Electrotherapy and Electrophysiologic Testing. Williams & Wilkins, Baltimore, 1989, p 101.

Credits

Class Activity 8, Current Density and Class Activity 9, Identification of Motor Points adapted from Starkey, C: Therapeutic Modalities for Athletic Trainers. FA Davis, Philadelphia, 1993.

Class Activity 10, Manual Determination of Stimulation Sites, adapted from Berlant, SR: Method of determining optimal stimulation sites for transcutaneous electrical nerve stimulation. Phys Ther 64:924, 1984.

The case studies were supplied by Susan Foreman, MS, ATC, PT.

Photographs by Jodie Humphrey, ATC, PT.